The █████████████████ ries

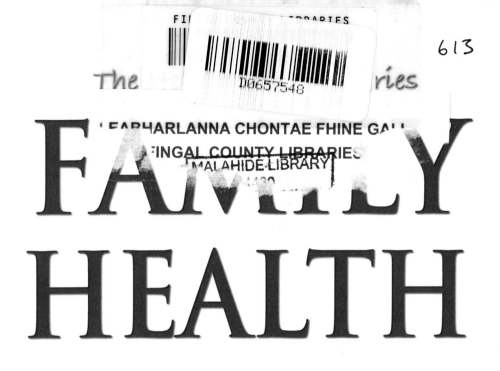

FAMILY
HEALTH

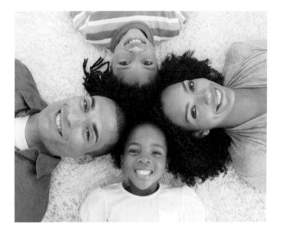

This is a **FLAME TREE** book
First published in 2010

Publisher and Creative Director: Nick Wells
Commissioning Editor: Polly Prior
Project Editor: Catherine Taylor
Copy Editor: Susan Aldridge
Art Director: Mike Spender
Layout Design: Dave Jones
Digital Design and Production: Chris Herbert
Picture Research: Kayla Yurick
Proofreader: Tony Phillips
Indexer: Helen Snaith

This edition first published 2010 by
FLAME TREE PUBLISHING
Crabtree Hall, Crabtree Lane
Fulham, London SW6 6TY
United Kingdom

www.flametreepublishing.com

Flame Tree is part of the Foundry Creative Media Co. Ltd
© 2010 this edition the Foundry Creative Media Company

ISBN 978-1-84786-706-3

A CIP record for this book is available from the British Library upon request.

Printed in China

All pictures are courtesy of Shutterstock and © the following photographers:
1 & 221, 78, 102, 202 Sean Prior; 4 & 16 Kzenon; 5b & 86 Alexander Raths; 5t & 54 Yulia Popkova; 6b & 152 Losevsky Pavel; 6t & 116, 7b & 222, 138 kristian sekulic;
7t & 180 Seti; 8 & 70, 126 Johnny Habell; 9r & 87br & 101r Teresa Kasprycka; 9l & 96 fred goldstein; 10 & 19 michaeljung; 11 & 69 Käfer photo; 12 & 95 Steven Frame;
13b & 172b Buhantsov Alexey; 13t & 121b SergeyPopov; 14 & 179, 77t, 110, 236 Andresr; 15 & 239b photobank.kiev.ua; 17br & 24 Elena Elisseeva; 18c courtyardpix;
18bl, 18br Morgan Lane Photography; 18cb Gertan; 18tr Karen Struthers; 18tl Krzysztof Slusarczyk; 20 Jaroslaw Grudzinski; 21 abimages; 22 Objectif MC; 23 studio 58; 25 Joerg Beuge;
26, 159 Dean Mitchell; 27 Dan Crown; 28 Dmitri Melnik; 31, 63 Photosani; 32 Olena Sokalska; 33 PeJo; 34 Roman Sigaev; 35 Wallenrock; 36 Anklav; 37t Akbudak Rimma; 37b & 170 Piotr
Marcinski; 39t TranceDrumer; 39b Zurijeta; 40 Zenphotography; 41 Arne Pastoor; 42 Phase4Photography; 43, 66, 94, 217 Lasse Kristensen; 45 krivenko; 46 Evgeny Tomeev; 48 Zholobov
Vadim; 49 Dmitri Mihhailov; 51 Darren Baker; 52 Phil Date; 53, 174t Studio 1One; 56 Jack Cronkhite; 58 & 55br Pinkcandy; 60 Marin; 62 Gemenacom; 68 metrmetr; 71 mashe; 72 Steinhagen
Artur; 74 Sorin Popa; 75 dean bertoncelj; 77b, 148, 169, 174b, 206 Monkey Business Images; 79 Robyn Mackenzie; 80 DUSAN ZIDAR; 81 Stephen Gibson; 82 D7INAMI7S; 83 Reggie Lavoie;
84, 89, 185, 229 Ilya Andriyanov; 90 Paul Vinten; 92 Bayanova Svetlana; 98 Yuris Schulz; 99 Magone; 103 pzAxe; 107 Stephen Mcsweeny; 109 Michael C. Gray; 111 mihalec; 117br Carlos E.
Santa Maria; 118 carroteater; 119 sarah johnson; 120 Sascha Burkard; 121t kenxro; 122 ukrphoto; 123 Olga OSA; 124 OlegD; 125, 226 prism68; 127 Donna Cuic; 128 Ruslan Kudrin; 130l
Miroslav Tolimir; 130r Tyler Olson; 131 EuToch; 132 Alon Brik; 133 Alexander Kalina; 134 John Sartin; 135 Voronin76; 137 Bernd Jürgens; 139 Juriah Mosin; 140, 231 aceshot1; 143 ampyang;
145 sergei telegin; 146 Udo Kröner; 147 ducu59us; 150t Istvan Csak; 150b, 177 Rudyanto Wijaya; 153br & 155 paul prescott; 154 arenacreative; 156 Amihays; 157 Elnur; 160 Marta
Tobolova; 163, 176 beerkoff; 164 Kesu; 165 LianeM; 166 Cagri Oner; 168, 223br & 251 vadim kozlovsky; 171 David Davis; 172t Crystal Kirk; 181br & 189 Golden Pixels LLC; 182 Gelpi;
184, 239t Suzanne Tucker; 186 Yanick Vallée; 188 ruzanna; 191 Vladislav Gajic; 193 MANDY GODBEHEAR; 195 photobunny; 196 Stacy Barnett; 198 Supri Suharjoto; 199 Tracy Whiteside;
200, 210 John McLaird; 204 Thomas M Perkins; 208 Balefire; 209 Gorilla; 212 N J Price; 213 Janaka Dharmasena; 214 Lisa A. Svara; 215 Christy Thompson; 218 Perkus; 220 Kuttelvaserova;
225b hkannn; 225t Laura Hart; 228 inginsh; 230 ENVY; 233 siamionau pavel; 235 Charles B. Ming Onn; 237 Radomir JIRSAK; 241 Ronald Sumners; 243t Christopher Futcher;
243b Edw; 244 Artix Studio; 245 comosaydice; 246 maxstockphoto; 247 studio BM; 248 tomashko

The Helping Hand Series

FAMILY
HEALTH

THE ESSENTIAL GUIDE TO DIET, MEDICINE & WELLBEING

**JO WATERS &
MARTINE GALLIE**

Consultant Editor: DR DAVID EDWARDS

**FLAME TREE
PUBLISHING**

Contents

Maintaining a healthy lifestyle is the first defence against illness, beginning with a well-balanced diet; so this section gives advice on how to achieve optimum nutrition, considering different groups' specific dietary requirements. Information is also provided on why and how to avoid cigarettes, drugs, too much alcohol and stress, along with how to sleep well and benefit from the relationships in your life.

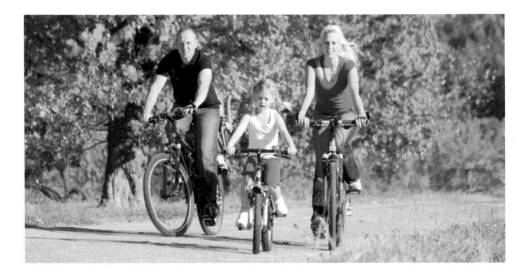

Head & Neck Health 54

Your head and neck house many organs and surfaces, inside and out, that are susceptible to illness. Your brain, and by extension your nervous system, can be attacked by conditions from epilepsy to Parkinson's disease, while your mental wellbeing can be diminished by psychological problems such as depression or eating disorders. This is not to mention the more obvious and common disorders that we can suffer in the ear, nose and throat, as well as the mouth and eyes – all are dealt with here.

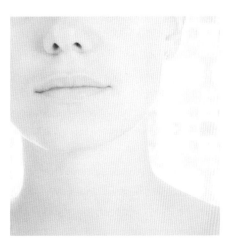

Chest & Abdominal Health 86

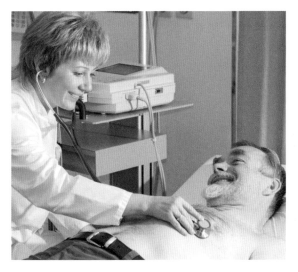

This part of your body contains most of your vital organs, which all have specific jobs to do in keeping you healthy. Here we look at what can go wrong with the chest, heart and lungs (from bronchitis to angina), the digestive system (from heartburn to appendicitis) and the urinary tract and liver (from cystitis to cirrhosis). We also discuss the problems that can occur with your back, whether it is general back pain or sciatica, and how to take better care of it.

Whole Body Health

People forget that their skin is one of the most important organs of their body – protecting them from all manner of foreign bodies and healing itself when it is injured. Even if we take good care of our skin, we may still suffer from conditions such as acne or eczema, so we provide lots of advice here. Equally our blood and circulation, and bones, muscles and joints are whole-body systems that are potentially vulnerable to illness and injury. We also deal here with the hands and feet, the immune system, the metabolism (diabetes) and sexual health.

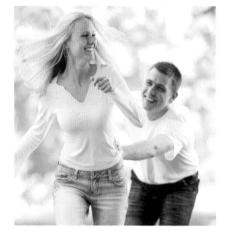

Men & Women's Health

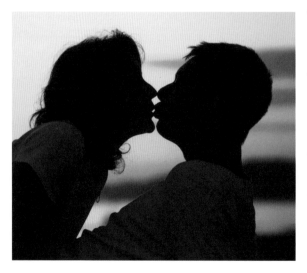

This section discusses the many health concerns and problems that are specific to each gender (or tend to be more relevant to one or the other), such as fertility, hormonal and sexual health and certain types of cancers. Classic issues for men, for example, are baldness, erection and prostate problems and hernias, while women can suffer from polycystic ovary syndrome or cervical cancer, and need tips on pregnancy health, for instance.

Children, like men and women, have specific health needs and concerns, and these change over the different stages of a child's life, from babyhood through to puberty and adolescence. So this section is structured accordingly, starting with advice on their first year, such as how to deal with a colicky or teething baby. Then learn about the various potential conditions of childhood, from head lice and chickenpox to asthma and ADHD. Finally, advice is provided on coping with teenagers, their illnesses and neuroses.

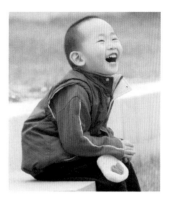

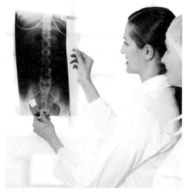

You never know when you may be in a situation when having learnt some of the essential emergency first aid procedures may help save someone's life. This book provides initial education on how to assess someone's condition – if they have just collapsed for example – and how to put them in the recovery position and attempt resuscitation if necessary. There is also further information on how to deal swiftly with injuries and conditions such as burns, bleeding, suspected broken bones and strains, choking, allergic reactions and poisoning.

Foreword

Traditionally the bedrock of self-care for health matters has rested within the family. Usually this source of folk knowledge came from the mother or grandmother, who either had seen or heard of someone who had suffered from the particular ailment in question. However, this status quo has crumbled in recent years for various reasons. Society has changed, with an increasing number of family units breaking up, leaving the carer or sufferer of the complaint unsupported. Increased mobility has resulted in the more experienced relative being separated by distance, sometimes countries apart, from the less knowledgeable and understandably concerned younger family member.

The internet, whilst being a huge knowledge base, can also present the browser with misinformation, manipulating signs and symptoms in order to promote online sales of drugs or boost attendance at some 'dodgy' private clinic.

There is, therefore, still a need for a quick, easy-to-access, means of finding out more about medical matters, whether they be lifestyle issues, more specific queries or, for example, questions regarding embarrassing problems that you might not want to discuss with a friend or family member.

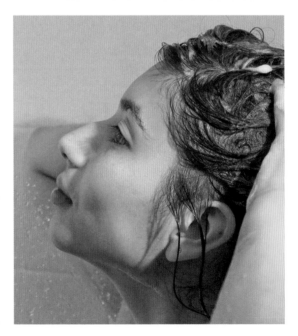

Family Health is an easy-to-read, informative book about day-to-day medical conditions, dietary and lifestyle issues. Each chapter is a signpost for speedy reference, with simple, clear text and no use of 'jargonese'! For some readers who want to know more about themselves it will be a fascinating read from start to finish; whilst for others it will be 'on call' ready to spring into action when the need arises. It will inform them as to what they can do to help themselves but, more importantly for some problems, assist and guide them as to whether they should be seeking expert medical attention.

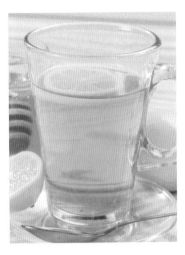

Family Health is not about replacing the expertise of a healthcare professional, in particular your family doctor. Neither is it proposing to make the experienced family member redundant should you be fortunate enough to possess one. Indeed it would seem to be an ideal gift for parents to give their offspring when they leave home or for proud grandparents to present to their newly born grandchild instead of yet another cuddly toy or woolly socks!

I welcome this addition to the household bookshelf.

Dr David Edwards

Introduction

Keeping your family healthy is an ongoing job. And trying to maintain a healthy lifestyle so that health problems don't develop in the first place is a good place to start. It's impossible to live on a diet of takeaways, fizzy drinks and cigarettes and expect to stay healthy. Being informed is vital, too, and so is knowing when it's time to call the doctor. In Family Health you'll find all the information you need to make the right health decisions for your family.

Keeping the Family Healthy

We are bombarded with health messages from all sides these days. Often it's not lack of information that stops us staying fit and healthy, it's having the time and motivation.

The trick is to set clear, realistic goals for you and your family. Rather than going straight from no exercise at all to a 30-minute run each day, start with 10-minute walks and build up from there. Try to make changes that you can sustain in the long term, too. Instead of cutting out alcohol altogether then falling off the wagon with a crash three days later, perhaps set aside two alcohol-free days each week. Write down your healthy-living goals and stick them on the fridge to remind you.

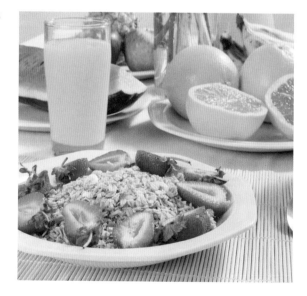

Be creative about how you encourage healthy habits. Simply telling children that they have to eat five portions of fruit and vegetables a day is unlikely to work. You're more likely to interest them in eating healthily if you involve them in shopping and cooking. Or have a competition to see who can invent the most delicious smoothie.

It helps to see healthy living as a team activity. If you keep fit and eat healthily, it's perfectly reasonable to have the same expectations of the rest of the family. Equally, there is no point in encouraging your partner or kids to be more active when you spend most of your life on the sofa. Encourage each other. It's far easier to change bad habits when you do it together than when you go it alone.

In this book, as well as tips on how to lead a healthy lifestyle, you'll also find detailed chapters about the different parts of your body. There are only a few bits and pieces – tonsils, adenoids, appendix and gallbladder – that we can happily manage without. Everything else has a crucial part to play and needs to be kept in good working order. We'll show you how.

Head and Neck

These house the brain and the top of the spinal cord. The head is also the seat of four of our five senses: smell, taste, sight and hearing. This book covers all the main disorders that affect the brain, from physical disorders, such as Parkinson's disease, to mental ones like bipolar disorder. Learn the symptoms and find out who's most at risk. You'll also find advice and tips on health problems affecting the eyes, ears, nose and mouth.

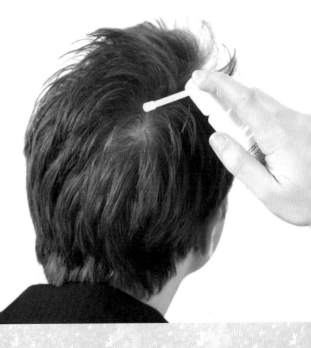

Chest and Abdominal Areas

Your chest is home to your heart and lungs and their health is essential to your overall wellbeing. Smoking is the biggest enemy of both, so giving up is a vital part of staying fit and healthy. Eating a healthy diet, getting some exercise, and keeping an eye on your alcohol intake will also go a long way to keeping your heart and lungs happy.

Most of us take our backs for granted. But back problems are common and can be distressing and debilitating. It really pays to look after your back and keep wear and tear to a minimum. Turn to pages 95–97 for tips on how to keep your back and spine in good working order.

Our digestive system, meanwhile, is one of the busiest areas of our bodies. It is permanently in motion breaking down the food we eat and disposing of what's not needed. A healthy diet that's rich in fibre can help to ward off potential problems like constipation and diverticular disease. Drinking plenty of fluids will not only help with digestion, it will help to keep your urinary tract free from infections, too. Your urinary tract performs the vital role of extracting a waste matter called urea from your blood stream and excreting it from the body. Sadly it's all too prone to infections, especially in women. Find out how to avoid them on pages 108–09.

Whole Body

We also take a look at all the other ailments that can affect our bodies, from dermatitis to arthritis to sexually transmitted infections. You'll find guidance on how to treat minor illnesses at home and advice on when to see your doctor. All the latest treatments are outlined and so are the symptoms to watch out for.

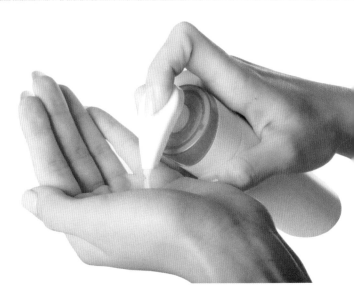

Men and Women

Men and women obviously share many of the same health problems. But differences in our physiologies also lead to gender-specific ailments. Men have particular issues relating to their sex organs and male hormones, such as enlarged prostates and testicular cancer. Women, on the other hand, have a different set of problems relating to their menstrual cycle and childbearing, including heavy periods and urinary incontinence.

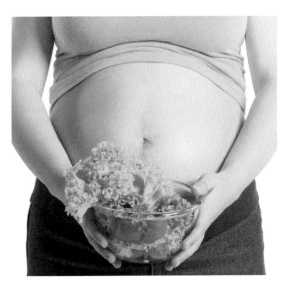

Sometimes there is simply no explanation for the differences in the conditions that affect men and women. No one knows why, for example, thyroid conditions are more common in women. And the reasons that high blood pressure tends to affect men at an earlier age than women are still not fully understood.

But perhaps the most significant difference between men and women as far as our health goes is the fact that women are better at seeking medical help for their problems. Men are generally more reluctant to see their doctors, preferring to ignore potentially worrying symptoms. Often it's their female partner who has to nag them into seeing a doctor. This book covers all the potentially dangerous symptoms that men need to look out for. If you recognize them in yourself, take your courage in your hands and get down to your local surgery.

The Early Years

During the baby and toddler years, when the immune system is still maturing, infections like gastroenteritis, chickenpox and colds will keep you busy with the thermometer and infant paracetamol. When your little one is ill, his sleeping and feeding patterns may well be disrupted as well. That means the added stress of sleepless nights and worries about whether or not he's getting all the nourishment he needs.

The school years bring new delights, such as head lice and threadworms. Thankfully, the more serious conditions that parents tend to worry about, such as meningitis, are rare, but it's still wise to know the symptoms. Hormone-related conditions like acne and body odour often arrive with the teenage years. These problems may not be medical emergencies, but need to be taken seriously because of the damage they can do to a teenager's fragile self-confidence.

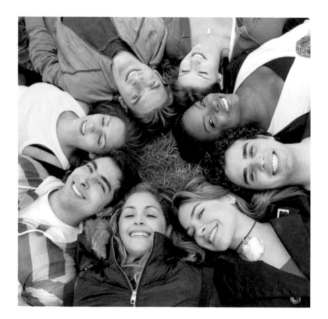

As parents we tend to fret over our children's health more than our own. To some degree this is wise. When children get ill they do tend to deteriorate faster than adults, so it makes sense to be watchful and cautious. The good news is that, with appropriate treatment, children also have an amazing ability to bounce back from illnesses – even quite serious ones – in a way that adults don't.

In an Emergency

It's a cliché to say it, but none of us ever expects to have to deal with an emergency in the home. The truth is that more accidents and emergencies happen in the home than anywhere else. Children under the age of five and people over the age of 65 are particularly vulnerable, and most injuries are due to falls. Other common accidents in the home include accidental poisonings and burns.

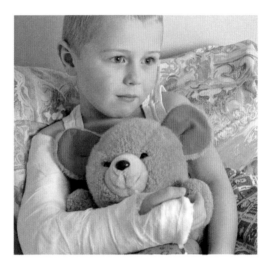

That's why this book has a whole chapter covering all the basic first aid you'll ever need in an emergency. Take the time to look through it and arm yourself with information that could save the life of a loved one.

A Final Word...

One last, important point: this book is not a substitute for a visit to your doctor. You know your body – and your children's bodies – better than anyone else. If you aren't sure whether something needs medical attention, or if you only have a hunch that it does, go and get it checked out. That is what your family doctor is there for. He or she will be glad to examine you and reassure you, and you'll have the peace of mind of knowing that all is well.

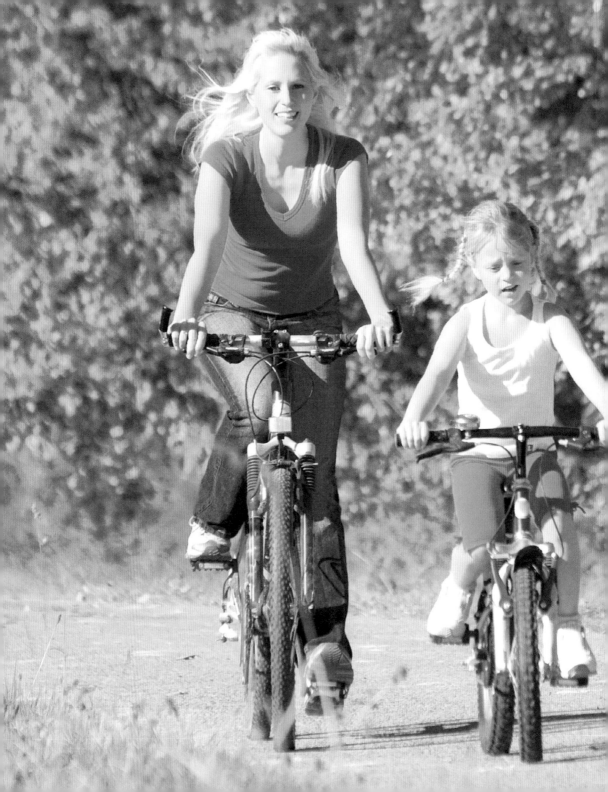

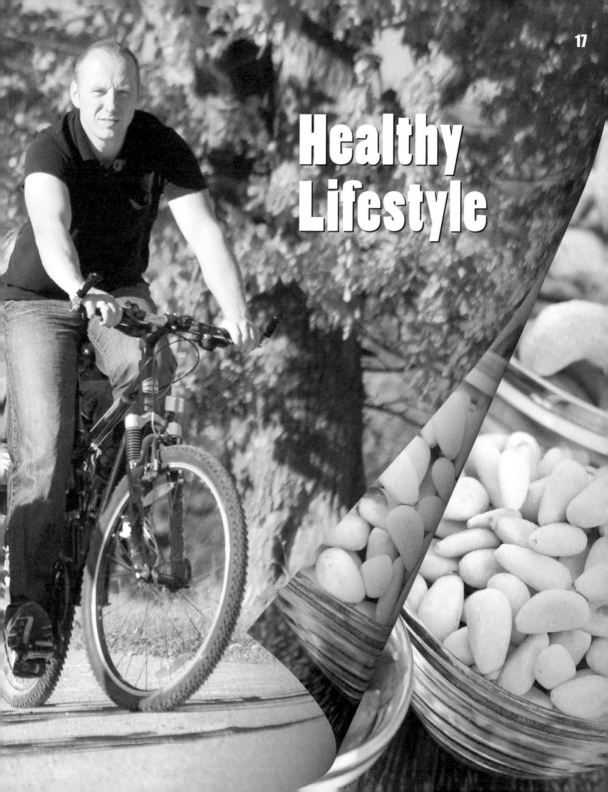

Healthy Lifestyle

Nutrition

It's a cliché, but you are what you eat. Our bodies function better and develop fewer faults if they are given the right fuel in the right amounts. There's a wealth of medical research out there now which suggests that many common conditions such as heart disease, strokes, type 2 diabetes, osteoporosis, tooth decay and a third of all cancers, are diet and lifestyle-related.

What Makes a Healthy Diet?

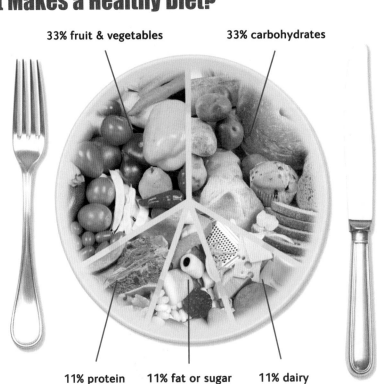

33% fruit & vegetables   33% carbohydrates

11% protein   11% fat or sugar   11% dairy

You need to eat a wide range of foods, including fruit and vegetables, carbohydrates, protein, fat, fibre and dairy products and limit your calorie intake to 1,940 a day if you're a woman and 2,550 for men – remember that this can vary based on age, height, weight and activity: for those with sedentary lifestyles who get little exercise this is the maximum to maintain weight. Calorie intakes for children vary according to their age and weight. Around a third of your daily intake should come from fruit and vegetables, one third from carbohydrates such as rice, pasta and potatoes and then around 11 per cent each from protein (meat, eggs and beans), high fat/sugary foods and milk and dairy products. The illustration on the left helps you visualize these proportions.

Base Your Meals on Starchy Carbohydrates

Carbohydrates include bread, pasta, rice, potatoes and cereals. Although they have a reputation for being fattening, they are much less dense in calories than fats and gram for gram they contain around half the calories. They're good for energy, B vitamins, fibre and calcium, in particular, and whole-grain carbohydrates take longer to digest so help you feel fuller for longer and also contain more nutrients.

Avoid Fatty Meat and Choose Leaner Cuts

Meat is a good source of protein, but try to avoid eating too much fatty red meat as it contains saturated fat which can clog up your arteries and lead to heart disease. Choose leaner cuts or white meat such as chicken or turkey which is lower in fat. Limit the amount of fatty processed meats you eat too, such as sausages, pâtés and cooked meats like salami.

Eat at Least Five Portions of Fruit and Vegetables a Day

These are packed with vitamins and minerals, low in calories and high in fibre so tick all the right boxes for good health. Fresh, frozen, canned and dried types all count, as does one glass of juice a day. Aim to eat a wide variety of different coloured fruit and veg too (think purple beetroot, orange carrots, red peppers, greens, yellow sweetcorn) – that way you'll ensure you get a wider range of vitamins and nutrients.

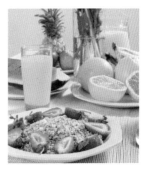

Top Tip

If you're pregnant, planning a pregnancy or breastfeeding, limit oily fish consumption to no more than two portions a week and avoid marlin, shark and swordfish completely because of their higher mercury content. High levels of mercury can affect a baby's development. Visit www.eatwell.gov.uk for more information.

Eat More Fish

Aim to eat at least two portions of fish a week, including one portion of oily fish such as mackerel, herring, fresh tuna, or sardines. They're rich in omega-3 fatty acids which can help protect you from heart disease and may be helpful in reducing the symptoms of other inflammatory illnesses such as rheumatoid arthritis. Omega-3 fatty acids may also help prevent depression and preserve cognitive function.

Avoid Too Much Sugar

Sugar, sugary foods and drinks are calorie-dense, so too many of them can result in weight gain and they're 'empty' calories too, with no added nutritional value. Sugar also attacks tooth enamel. Check sugar content on processed food labels such as jams and biscuits – a low-sugar food will have less than 5 g of sugars per 100 g and a high-sugar food will have more than 15 g of sugar per 100 g.

Know Your Fats

Fats are high in calories, but not all types of fat are bad for you. There are three main types:

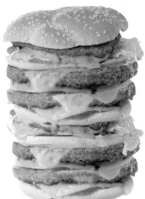

- **Saturated fats**: These are associated with clogged arteries and heart disease. They should make up no more than a third of your total fat intake. They are found in red meat, processed foods, butter, lard, cakes and biscuits, full-fat dairy food etc.
- **Trans-fats**: These are vegetable oils which have been processed (by partial hydrogenation) to make them hard. They are used in many processed foods such as cakes, biscuits, pastries and some ready meals. Keep these fats to a minimum.

Unsaturated fats: Found in plant foods such as seeds, fruit, vegetables and nuts, these can be divided into two groups: polyunsaturated fats (from sunflower, soya and corn) and monounsaturated fats (found in olive oil and rapeseed oil). Polyunsaturated fats have cholesterol-lowering properties and monounsaturated fats are the main staple of the so-called Mediterranean diet (olive oil, tomatoes, fruit and vegetables, red wine and oily fish), which has been associated with a lower incidence of heart disease.

Don't Forget Dairy Products

Milk is a great source of fat, calcium, vitamins and other minerals; choose semi-skimmed or skimmed to save on calories and reduce the saturated fat content, (children under two should be given full-fat milk). Hard cheeses such as Cheddar are good sources of calcium but also contain saturated fat so use sparingly (grate instead of slice for instance) or choose lower fat cheeses such as cottage cheese.

Eat No More Than 6 g of Salt a Day

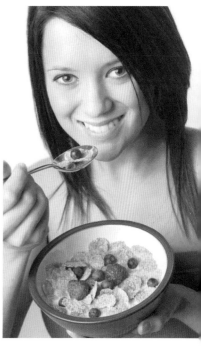

Too much salt can lead to high blood pressure which puts you at higher risk of stroke and heart attack. We're all eating far too much of it (an average of 12 g a day according to some estimates). Recommended daily salt intake for children varies according to age from less than 1 g a day in breast milk up to one year, gradually increasing to 5 g a day by age seven to 10 and 6 g at age 11 to 16. To visualize: 6 g of salt is about a teaspoonful – and that's the maximum!

 Avoid eating too many salty processed foods: Ready meals, tinned soups, Chinese takeaways, gravy powder and pizza are all loaded with hidden salt; also check the salt content on breakfast cereals, biscuits and bread.

 Cook from scratch wherever you can: That way you control the salt content.

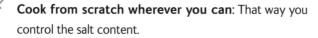

Vitamins and Minerals

Your body needs a wide range of foods containing all the vitamins, minerals and trace elements in order to function healthily.

The Vitamins

These are essential nutrients which are needed for a number of specific processes in the body. Some vitamins are fat-soluble which means that the body can store them for future use (such as vitamins A, D, E and K) and others are water-soluble (vitamins B6, B12, C, biotin, pantothenic acid, riboflavin and thiamine),

which means they cannot be stored and you need to eat them every day. Vitamins can also be damaged or destroyed by cooking, heat and exposure to air, so try and eat fruit and vegetables soon after you buy them or use frozen or dried versions and lightly steam vegetables rather than boil away all the goodness.

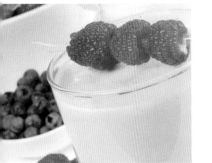

- **Vitamin A:** Good for healthy skin, immunity and boosting vision in poor light. It's also needed for healthy functioning of cells that line the respiratory tract and gastro-intestinal tract. It's found in cheese, eggs, milk, fortified margarines and yoghurts. Avoid eating liver and liver pâté and other vitamin A rich foods in pregnancy, as they can prove dangerous to foetal development.
- **Thiamine (vitamin B1):** Needed for healthy nerves and muscle tissue and also to help release energy from food. It's added to some breakfast cereals and found in pork, vegetables, milk, dried fruit, eggs, wholegrains and breads.
- **Riboflavin (vitamin B2):** Vital for healthy skin and nervous system and helps produce

red blood cells. It is used to fortify breakfast cereals and is found in milk, eggs, mushrooms and rice.

 Pantothenic acid (vitamin B5): Helps release energy from food and helps the body deal with stress. It's found in meat and vegetables including eggs, broccoli, beef, chicken and potatoes.

 Vitamin B6: Needed for production of haemoglobin in red blood cells to carry oxygen around the body and also releasing energy from protein and carbohydrate in foods, as well as speeding up many other chemical reactions in the body. You'll find it in pork, chicken, turkey, cod, whole-grain cereals, eggs, vegetables, soya beans, peanuts, milk, potatoes and fortified breakfast cereals. It is estimated around one in 5 women and one in five elderly people may be deficient in vitamin B6.

Biotin (vitamin B7): Helps the body turn food into energy. It also keeps hair and nails healthy. Good sources include kidney, eggs, nuts and dried fruit.

Folic acid or folate (vitamin B9): Needed to form healthy red blood cells and has an important role to play in preventing the neural tube defect spina bifida (*see* page 172). It's found in green vegetables such as broccoli and asparagus, peas, bananas, brown rice and fortified breakfast cereals.

Vitamin B12: Prevents a form of anaemia (pernicious anaemia *see* page 132) and is believed to help prevent depression and nerve pain. It's found in offal, sardines, eggs, meat and cheese and is also used to fortify breakfast cereals.

Vitamin C: Used throughout the body it boosts immunity, speeds up wound healing, may help the body to absorb iron from foods and generally protects cells and helps keep them healthy. It's found in fruit and vegetables, especially peppers, broccoli, Brussels sprouts, oranges and kiwi fruit.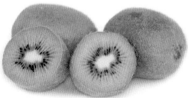

Vitamin D: Known as the 'sunshine' vitamin as your body synthesizes it from sunlight. Vitamin D is also added to some fortified breakfast cereals and is found in oily fish such as herring, salmon and tuna. It's needed for healthy bones and teeth and may slow down the progression of the brittle-bone disease osteoporosis. Too little vitamin D can cause rickets in children.

Vitamin E: Acts as an antioxidant – helping to neutralize or destroy free radicals (unstable oxygen molecules which cause damage to cells – which can lead to disease). They're found in soy, corn and olive oils, plus nuts, seeds and wheat germ.

 Vitamin K: Promotes blood clotting and boosts healing of wounds and is also needed for strong bones and is believed to play a role in preventing osteoporosis. It's found in leafy green vegetables such as spinach and broccoli.

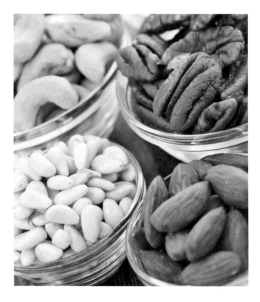

Minerals and Trace Elements

There are more than 60 different minerals in the body and some are needed (often only in minute quantities known as trace elements) for a variety of vital chemical processes. Here are some of the most important ones:

 Calcium: Needed for strong bones and teeth. It's found in dairy products, leafy green vegetables and bony fish such as pilchards/sardines. It is also added to bread.

 Magnesium: Essential for converting energy from food plus healthy nerve and muscle function. It's found in wholegrains, nuts and dark-green leafy vegetables.

 Potassium: Needed to regulate heart beat and blood pressure and conduct nerve impulses. Fresh fruit and vegetables, particularly bananas, are good sources.

Did You Know?

You need to expose your arms and face to sunlight (outdoors) without sunscreen for 15 minutes a day for your body to make enough vitamin D?

Top Tip

Did you know if you're a smoker you may need higher levels of vitamin C and other antioxidants? Cigarette smoke stimulates the production of free radicals (unstable oxygen molecules) that cause cell damage.

- **Phosphorus:** Helps store energy in cells and is also needed to interact with calcium to build strong bones and teeth. It's found in meats, fish, poultry and dairy products.
- **Sodium and chloride (salt):** Found in all tissues and helps regulate fluid balance in the body. Chloride is needed to make stomach juices to digest foods. Too much salt is associated with high blood pressure (hypertension) and increases the risk of heart attacks and strokes.
- **Zinc:** An 'all rounder' mineral needed to maintain a healthy immune system, improve skin conditions, boost sex hormones and thyroid production and digest food. It's found in protein sources such as meat, eggs, brazil nuts, almonds and seafood (especially oysters).
- **Selenium:** Trace mineral which has an antioxidant effect to protect cells against damage from 'free radicals' that otherwise result in diseases such as cancer and heart disease. It is also needed in the production of thyroid hormones which regulate metabolism and is important for the immune system and reproduction. You can get selenium from nuts, meat and fish.

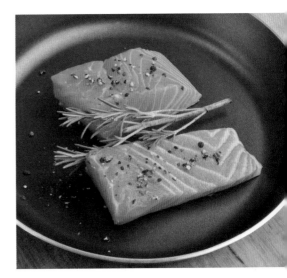

- **Iron:** Essential for making red blood cells (haemoglobin) which transport oxygen around the body. Red meat is the best source but you can also get it from dried fruit and leafy greens such as spinach.

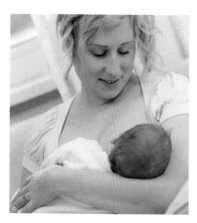

Different Life-stage Requirements

Each stage of your life will pose different nutritional requirements. Here's what you need to eat when:

Babies up to Six Months

The best nutrition for babies is breast milk – expertly formulated by nature to give your growing baby everything she or he needs. If breastfeeding isn't for you, infant formulae (powdered baby milks) are a good second best. Do bear in mind, however, that breastfeeding also has the following advantages:

 Breastfeeding is free: It's available instantly on demand without the hassle of sterilizing and warming-up bottles.

Breastfeeding expends energy: Since it uses up to 500 of your daily calorie intake, breastfeeding is great for helping you shed those post-pregnancy pounds.

Six–12 Months

By six months your baby will begin moving onto solid foods (a process known as weaning), starting with baby rice, puréed vegetables and fruit, before progressing to 'finger food' he/ she can hold and feed themselves – although not usually until towards the end of their first year. The more solid food your baby eats the less milk they will drink. Their calorie needs will depend on their weight so check with your health visitor or family doctor.

Toddlers

Some dos and don'ts on feeding your toddler:

Provide small calorie-packed meals: Toddlers have high energy needs but can't manage large portions

Did You Know?

Breast milk protects your baby against ear infections, gastro-intestinal infections, chest infections, urine infection, childhood diabetes, eczema, obesity and asthma.

in the same way that an adult can, so focus on giving them small but healthy high energy snacks which are also packed with vitamins and nutrients, including full-fat milk, cheese, yoghurts, fruit and vegetables, meat and eggs.

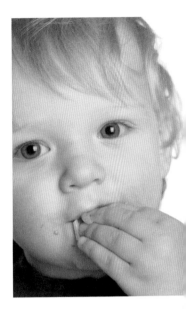

 Go easy on wholemeal bread, rice and pasta: Don't overload on these as they can be harder for them to digest.

 Switch to semi–skimmed milk: Change to this after two years – it contains the same amount of calcium (needed for healthy bones and teeth – see page 138) as full-fat milk.

Avoid sugary drinks: Keep these to a minimum to protect against tooth decay and encourage them to drink fruit juice at mealtimes rather than between meals – even better, encourage them to drink water instead.

Five to Teens

Most children should be eating the same foods as the rest of the family by age five.

Make sure they eat breakfast: Children who eat breakfast have better concentration levels at school so make sure they eat a breakfast based around slow-release carbohydrates (such as porridge, wholemeal toast etc.), to keep their energy levels up to lunchtime.

Make them healthy packed lunches: Don't include too many high-fat/sugary foods – include a protein-based sandwich on wholemeal bread, two portions of fruit or chopped raw vegetables, yoghurt or small piece of cheese.

Watch out for E numbers/artificial additives: Avoid giving your child too many foods with these. This is especially important if they suffer from Attention Deficit Hyperactivity Disorder (ADHD). A study commissioned by the UK's Food Standards Agency published in 2007 found that if a child with ADHD had tartrazine (E102), Quionoline yellow (E104), Sunset yellow (E110), Carmisine (E122), Ponceasu 4 R (E124), Allura red (E129) and Sodium benzoate (E211) cut out of their diet, their behaviour improved.

- **Discourage eating junk food**: Eating too much junk food has also been associated with lower achievement at school.
- **Feed them fish**: Eating oily fish which contains omega-3 essential fatty acids may boost concentration and cognitive function.

Teenagers

Puberty is a time when the body grows rapidly and so energy needs increase.

- **Give them healthy snacks**: Teenagers have a tendency to 'graze', searching the fridge and kitchen cupboards for a quick energy-boosting snack. Snacking is fine – they're growing after all – but try and limit the amount of high-fat/high-sugar snacks they are consuming (eg: crisps, chocolate and sugary/fizzy drinks) and stock up with fresh fruit.
- **Don't let them skip breakfast**: Eating a slow-release carbohydrate-based breakfast such as wholemeal toast, or porridge, will help them feel fuller for longer and boost their concentration at school. Research studies have shown that combining protein (such as eggs) with carbohydrates can help you feel fuller for longer and help you control your weight.
- **Build up their bone density**: One in four teens have a calcium intake below the recommended level. Building up bone density before age 30 can help prevent the brittle-bone disease osteoporosis (it causes fractures in one in three older women and one in five men over 50). Encourage them to eat two to three portions of dairy food a day (think matchbox-sized slices of cheese, yoghurts, semi-skimmed milk on cereal) and stress the importance of weight-bearing exercise too.
- **Give teenage girls iron-rich foods**: Girls in their teens need iron-rich foods including red meat, dried fruits, eggs, baked beans, oily fish such as sardines and green leafy vegetables such as watercress, as menstrual bleeding can deplete their iron stores and lead to anaemia, causing tiredness and lethargy. They need 14.8 mg of iron a day (men need 8.7 mg a day).

Trying for a Baby

Eat a healthy diet based on a wide range of foods including five portions of fruit and vegetables, lean protein, two portions of oily fish a week, dairy products and carbohydrates. See the chapter on Women's Health for information on nutrition when pregnant or breastfeeding (pages 172–73).

- Stop smoking
- Stick to safe limits of alcohol (currently a maximum of two to three units of alcohol a day)
- Limit oily fish to no more than two portions of oily fish (mackerel, sardines and trout) a week
- Lose weight – it can boost your fertility if you are overweight

Did You Know?

All women trying for a baby or in the first three months of pregnancy should take a 400 mcg folic acid supplement. Taking folic acid in these crucial months can reduce the risk of a neural tube defect (spina bifida) by 75 per cent.

60 Plus

As you get older you generally become less active and need fewer calories, so you may find you'll need to eat less if you're going to avoid putting on weight in old age.

- **Eat plenty of fibre-rich foods**: These include oats, beans, lentils and wholegrain cereals. This helps to avoid constipation, a common problem as you get older, and boost intestinal health.
- **Get enough calcium**: This is found in dairy products, leafy green veg and fortified bread and helps maintain your bone density and prevent the brittle-bone disease osteoporosis, which affects one in three women and one in five older men.
- **Eat a prostate-friendly diet**: For older men, this will reduce your chances of developing prostate cancer. Just eating two cooked portions of tomatoes a week can cut your chances of developing prostate cancer by one third. The magic ingredient is a chemical called lycopene, which is also found in pink grapefruit, guava and papaya.

> ## Top Tip
>
> Switch to six healthy small meals and snacks a day rather than three big meals so you don't have to digest too much at one sitting.

☑ **Avoid eating too much saturated fat**: This is found in red meat, ready meals, cakes, pastries, sausages and other processed foods. It raises cholesterol in the blood and clogs the arteries and increases the risk of heart disease and stroke. Women need to be more aware of this after the menopause as their levels of the female sex hormone oestrogen drop and they lose the protection that this has given them up until this point.

☑ **Cut down on salt**: Salt raises blood pressure, so this is important because blood pressure rises as you get older and is a risk factor for stroke.

☑ **Get enough vitamin D**: Many older people, especially those who are housebound or who live in care homes – don't get enough exposure to sunlight to make sufficient vitamin D and may need supplements.

☑ **Eat iron-rich foods** (*see* page 28) to avoid developing iron-deficiency anaemia, which results in the production of less haemoglobin to carry oxygen around the blood in red blood cells.

☑ **Drink a small glass of red wine**: A small amount of alcohol daily may protect against heart disease in post menopausal women and men over 40. However, women have to balance these benefits against an increased risk of breast cancer that comes with drinking even one unit a day of alcohol. (For more on this *see* the section on alcohol, page 36.)

Eating to Prevent Disease

Certain foods are protective against specific diseases.

The Polymeal Diet

Researchers at Erasmus MC University in Rotterdam have devised a 'polymeal' of healthy ingredients, which they claim, if eaten daily could increase life expectancy by 4.8 years for women and by 6.6 years for men. It would also slash the risk of developing heart disease by 76 per cent. They suggest eating the following:

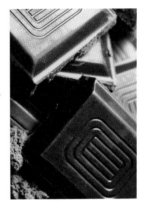

 Chocolate: Eat 100 g/3½ oz of dark chocolate a day to bring down blood pressure and reduce the risk of heart attacks by 21 per cent.

 Fruit: Eat 400 g/14 oz of fruit every day to reduce the risk by the same amount again.

 Wine: One 150 ml/¼ pint glass of wine a day (white or red, but red is better) can reduce cardiovascular disease by 32 per cent.

 Garlic and almonds: 2.7 g/¹⁄₁₀ oz of fresh garlic and 68 g/2½ oz of almonds a day will lower cholesterol.

 Oily fish: Four portions of 114 g/4 oz of oily fish (mackerel, herring or fresh tuna, for example) will reduce your risk of developing heart disease by 14 per cent.

Did You Know?

It's a myth that most cholesterol in blood comes from so-called high cholesterol foods like eggs and shellfish – most comes from saturated fat from foods such as red meat and processed foods.

The Portfolio Diet (Anti-Cholesterol)

The Portfolio Diet designed by Canadian academics at the University of Toronto has been shown to lower cholesterol by 30 per cent. It consists of four different key elements:

 Nuts: Aim to eat 30 g/1 oz a day (about 23 almonds). They're packed full of vegetable protein, fibre, heart-healthy monosaturated fats and vitamin E. Clinical trials have shown they have a beneficial effect on cholesterol.

 Soya Protein: Eating 50 g a day of soya protein is recommended. Found in soya milk, soya mince, soya beans, tofu and tempeh. It reduces production of cholesterol in the liver and increases the rate at which 'bad' low-density lipoprotein (LDL) cholesterol is removed from the blood. Use soya products as substitutes for meat or dairy milk and yoghurt or use tofu as a meat replacement in a stir-fry.

 Soluble fibre: Aim to eat 20 g daily. Even eating less than one ounce of soluble fibre per day has a positive effect on cholesterol. Found in oats, oatmeal, oat bran, barley, psyllium, beans, pulses, fruits and vegetables. Soluble fibre helps reduce LDL cholesterol by binding to fat in the diet.

 Plant Sterols: Eat 2 g daily. These are added to functional cholesterol-lowering foods such as spreads and yoghurts and found naturally in soya bean, corn, squash, vegetable oils and grains. They block cholesterol absorption in the gut.

The Anti-Cancer Diet

Eating an unhealthy diet can increase the risk of developing cancer by between 10 and 30 per cent in developed countries.

Did You Know?

Eating less red and processed meat could cut your cancer risk. The EPIC study found people who ate daily 80 g portions of processed meats increased their bowel cancer risk by a third compared to those who ate 20 g a day.

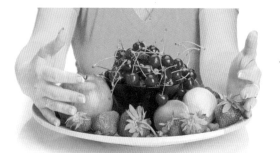

Go for a high fibre diet: Diets high in fibre can reduce the risk of bowel cancer by 25 to 40 per cent. That's according to the European Prospective Investigation into Cancer and Nutrition (EPIC) study – a six-year study of 520,000 people in 10 different European countries. However some studies from North America have not found the same association – but experts believe this is because Americans typically eat a diet much lower in fibre than Europeans.

Eat at least five portions of fruit and vegetables a day: Eating lots of fruit and vegetables can reduce the risk of dying from cancer, heart disease and diabetes by a quarter. Eating five a day also helps you keep to a healthy body weight and reduces the risk of developing cancers associated with obesity – including bowel, breast, kidney, womb and oesophageal cancers

Keeping to a Healthy Weight

Following a healthy diet will help keep you within a healthy weight range.

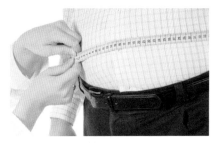

Do I Need to Lose Weight?

To check if you are in a healthy weight range for your height:

- **Calculate your Body Mass Index (BMI):** This is your weight in kilograms divided by your height in metres squared. Below 18.5 is underweight, between 18.5 and 24.9 is the ideal weight for your height, and 25–30 means you are classed as overweight, while 30–40 is classed as obese. A BMI of 40 is morbidly obese, which means your weight is a serious threat to your health. It is important to note, however, this calculation is not an accurate tool for very muscular people because muscle weighs more than fat.

- **Check your waist-to-hip ratio (WHR):** Weight gain around your waist (the classic apple shape) is linked to heart disease and circulatory problems. Measure your waist (abdominal) circumference and divide it by your hip circumference. If the figure is more than 0.85 for a woman and 0.9 for a man you have a higher risk of developing heart diseases. This ratio is much more significant than the BMI – for instance, people from ethnic groups such as south Asian, who are typically 'thinner' or have lower BMIs, may still have high WHRs and be at risk of heart disease. Irrespective of the ratio, women with a waist measurement of more than 32 inches and men who measure 37 inches or more are at greater risk of heart disease.

Count Calories

Stick to recommended calorie intake levels (*see* page 19), and adjust them according to how active you are.

Alcohol, Cigarettes and Drugs

Lifestyle factors such as drinking too much alcohol and smoking tobacco can have a detrimental effect on your health. They're just as important as diet and exercise when it comes to increasing your risk of developing such disease as cancer and high blood pressure.

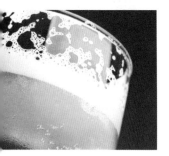

Alcohol

It's easy to get confused about whether alcohol is good or bad for you, as there is so much conflicting advice. With so many stronger types of wine and beer for sale in supermarkets and bars - it's also difficult to calculate exactly how many units of alcohol you're consuming. For instance if your daily glass of wine is a large one (250 ml) and the alcohol content is 12 per cent then one glass can contain as many as 2.5 units.

Small Amounts Can Be Good for Your Heart

Smallish amounts of alcohol (one or two units a day for women or three or four for men (see the tip box for definition of a unit) may offer some protection against heart disease. This is because alcohol raises levels of 'good' cholesterol (high density lipoprotein or HDL) which protects the arteries and also reduces the stickiness of the blood, cutting your risk of heart attack or stroke. These benefits only apply to men over 40 and post-menopausal women and the same effects can be achieved through exercise or following a healthy diet. However, if you don't drink already – no-one would advocate you take it up now just to protect your heart!

Did You Know?

Know your units: As a rough guide one unit of alcohol = 10 ml or 8 g of pure alcohol which equates to one small (125 ml) glass of wine, half a pint of beer or cider or one 25 ml measure of spirits.

Red Wine Trumps White Wine

There's some evidence that red wine may be best for you as it contains high levels of polyphenols, which have an antioxidant effect and can protect your arteries. Polyphenols are also found in foods such as grape juice and green tea – so you don't have to drink alcohol to get them.

The Dangers of Alcohol

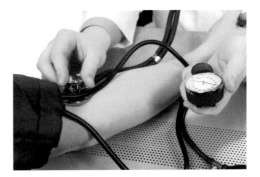

 Increased blood pressure: Too much alcohol can raise your blood pressure and enlarge your heart muscle. Men who drink more than four units a day and women who drink more than three units a day on a regular basis (a couple of times a week) may raise their blood pressure and increase their risk of heart attack or stroke. A heavy drinking session may lead to a condition called cardiomyopathy, where the heart muscle thickens and causes problems such as heart failure and disruptions in the heart rhythm.

 Increased breast cancer risk: The added complication for women is that even one unit of alcohol a day has been shown to raise the risk of breast cancer. The Million Woman Study published in the UK in 2009 has shown a statistically significant increase in cancer risk from just consuming one drink a day. It concluded that 13 per cent of all breast cancer cases can be attributed to low to moderate alcohol consumption.

 Other health problems: Too much alcohol can lead to problems such as depression, liver problems, reduced fertility, weight gain and forgetfulness.

Keep Within Safe Limits

The more alcohol you drink the more you damage your body, so stick to sensible amounts – not more than three to four units a day for a man and two to three units a day for women, a couple of times a week.

Cigarettes

You probably know tobacco causes lung cancer and a whole host of other health problems – including the lung disease emphysema, and chronic bronchitis. Most smokers want to give up but nicotine is highly addictive and it can be a difficult habit to quit.

Top Tip

If you do have a heavy 'binge' drinking session (and we're not advising you do!) give your body 48 hours to recover before you drink alcohol again.

Why Smoking is Bad for You (and Others)

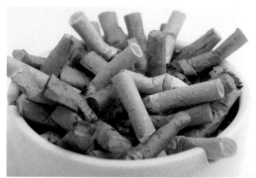

- **Lung cancer:** The link between smoking and lung cancer was discovered over 50 years ago. Ninety per cent of lung cancer cases are caused by smoking. Unfortunately most cases of lung cancer are not discovered until a late stage so survival rates are very low – just 27 per cent of people are still alive one year after diagnosis and seven per cent after five years. A sobering thought.

- **Ulcers and acid indigestion:** Smoking also increases your chances of developing a duodenal ulcer and acid indigestion.

- **Decreased fertility:** Chemicals in tobacco affect sperm quality and the lining of the womb.

- **Dangerous for your unborn baby:** If you're pregnant remember that when you inhale cigarette smoke it contains 4,000 chemicals, including carbon monoxide which can restrict your baby's oxygen and nutrient supply and affect growth. Babies born to smokers are more likely to be premature and have a low birth weight. Smoking can also increase the risk of miscarriage or stillbirth. Smoke inhaled by living with a partner who

smokes, affects the health of your unborn baby too.
Babies born to smokers are also at higher risk of cot
death (Sudden Infant Death Syndrome) or suffering
respiratory illnesses.

 Passive smoking: If your partner is a smoker you are
two to three times more likely to develop lung cancer
than a non-smoker.

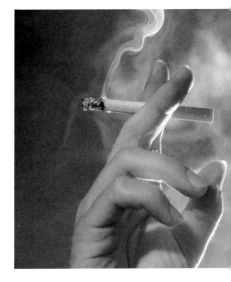

 Teeth and skin: Smokers often develop yellow teeth
and have a higher incidence of gum disease. Their skin
often appears thicker and ages quicker – this is
because smoking boosts the production of free
radicals – unstable oxygen molecules which can cause
cell damage.

Did You Know?

**It's never too late to give up smoking. You'll extend your life by 10 years
if you give up at the age of 30 and by three years if you give up at 60.**

Giving up Smoking

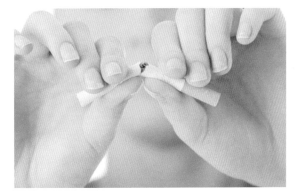

Get support: You're four
times more likely to succeed
at giving up smoking if you
get some professional help.
Ask your doctor about what
support and advice is available
locally. Some surgeries run

smoking cessation clinics and there are also schemes where you can get one to one counselling and telephone support.

- ✓ **Nicotine replacement therapy**: Your doctor can also prescribe nicotine replacement therapy (gums, patches, microtabs and nasal sprays) to help you deal with your craving.
- ✓ **Other drug therapies**: Drugs such as Bupropion Hydrochloride and Varenicline can help ease you through the transition period of withdrawal.
- ✓ **Hypnotherapy**: This has been shown to be helpful. Try CDs or see a qualified therapist.

Recreational Drugs

These drugs are illegal and include cannabis, cocaine, ecstasy, hallucinogenics and amphetamines. Even casual use can lead to health problems and in some cases addiction.

Cannabis

Cannabis is a commonly-used recreational drug. Most people perceive it is a 'soft' drug that helps them relax but one in 10 cannabis users also experience unpleasant reactions, including confusion, hallucinations, anxiety and paranoia. Research has also linked cannabis use with a higher risk of developing depression and mental illnesses such as schizophrenia.

- ✓ **Skunk**: Skunk is a type of cannabis which has a higher concentration of the psycho-active component – it is around two to three times stronger than the 'herbal' type cannabis that was available 30 years ago. It can induce extreme feelings of relaxation and elation but also anxiety attacks, projectile vomiting and a big increase in appetite.

Did You Know?

Smoking cannabis before the age of 16 makes you four times more likely to develop schizophrenia as an adult.

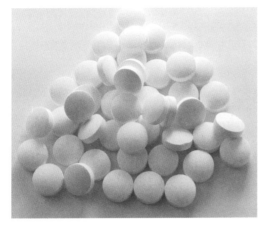

Ecstasy (or 'E's)

These became popular in the 1990s as a clubber's 'rave' drug which helped users stay awake and dance all night. The effects last about three to six hours and give an energy buzz and intensify colour and sound and make users lively and chatty. However, the drug has a dangerous side; it makes the heart beat faster, causes pupils to dilate and raises body temperature, increasing the chances of overheating and dehydration. Ecstasy has caused 200 deaths in the UK since 1996 and has caused dangerous reactions in people with asthma, epilepsy or a heart condition.

Amphetamines (Speed)

Amphetamines are a type of stimulant that people take to stay awake and feel alert. They also stop you feeling hungry, but are highly addictive. The 'high' is followed by a slow 'come down' during which time it can be difficult to relax or sleep. They can also put a strain on your heart and immune system and should be avoided by anyone with high blood pressure.

Cocaine

Cocaine is a highly addictive stimulant drug which can be inhaled or snorted as white powder or smoked as 'crack'. It gives a very intense high feeling – which lasts for between 10 and 30 minutes, depending on how it has been smoked or inhaled. Users say they feel on

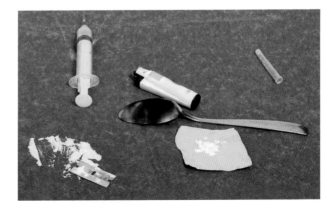

top of their game, but it can also induce panic attacks, fits or heart attacks and the high is usually followed by an equally intense low which can make people feel depressed and run down. Even casual use can soon lead to addiction.

Heroin

Heroin is an opiate made from morphine extracted from the opium poppy. It acts as a strong painkiller reducing physical and psychological pain and slows down body functioning. Users will experience a buzz after a few minutes. It causes intense cravings in the brain and is highly addictive. Deaths from overdose occur. Inhaling vomit may also be fatal as it can inhibit the cough reflex.

Top Tip

If you are a drug user, a number of charities and health-service support organizations can help you overcome your addiction. Try www.talktofrank.com as a first move.

Prescription and Over-the-counter Painkillers

Addiction to legal drugs – particularly headache pills and codeine-based medicines is a growing problem. If you suspect you are getting hooked talk to your doctor.

Stress and Relationships

Some pressure can be good for you in the short term; for example it helps motivate you to meet deadlines and you may perform better. However, in the long term stress can have toxic effects on the body. Meanwhile, relationship problems can be a major source of stress. So it's important for your health to keep your relationships strong.

Why Stress is Bad for You

When your body is stressed it releases chemicals including cortisol, adrenaline and noradrenaline – so-called 'fight or flight' hormones which help you up your game to take on challenges - or escape from them. Problems arise when you produce these chemicals and then are unable to use them up. A build up of adrenalin and noradrenaline can cause raised blood pressure, for instance, and cortisol prevents your immune system from functioning properly.

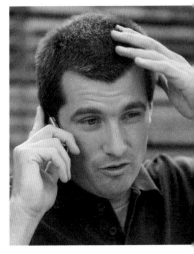

Symptoms of Stress

These can include:

- **Physical problems**: Such as chest pains, dizziness, breathlessness, sleep problems, diarrhoea and pins and needles.
- **Psychological difficulties**: Such as depression, anger, tearfulness, concentration problems and either an increase or decrease in appetite.

How to Manage Your Stress Levels

There are many ways to combat stress, starting first with working out the root causes and doing your best to address them.

Recognition and action: Recognize the signs of when you are becoming overloaded and take steps to ease off some of the pressure. If you're depressed, angry and tearful try and take a step back and look at what is triggering these feelings. If you are overloaded at work – talk to your boss about delegating or reorganizing your workload. If you are trying to juggle work with caring for children consider a part-time option and/or get your partner to share more of the domestic responsibilities. If you are overwhelmed by the needs of your children – ask for help from a friend or relative or even a charity that specialize in supporting families.

Ask your doctor for help: Stress is increasingly recognized as an important factor in your overall health. You may need medication such as sedatives, antidepressants, antihistamines or beta blockers to help treat your symptoms, or talking therapies (see tip box).

Learn to relax: It's important to be able to switch off from work or the pressure of caring for children, so try and carve out some time for yourself every day where you do something you enjoy. Try a soak in the bath with scented candles, a gym session, walk or run, reading a book or listening to a relaxation CD. Switch off your mobile and email and find some time to chill.

Try a herbal remedy: Rhodiola rosea root extract can give you extra support to deal with the symptoms of stress such as anxiety, exhaustion and depression and is available from pharmacies. Ginseng might also help but there is little medical evidence for this.

Top Tip

Talking therapies such as counselling or cognitive behavioural therapy (CBT) can help you deal with your feelings and see the pressures of the stresses and strains in your life in a different way. CBT in particular teaches you to reframe events in a positive way.

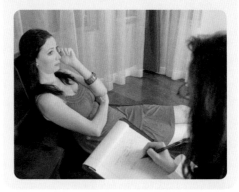

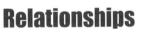 **Stay close to friends and family**: Maintain contact with friends and family who will support you – it's important you don't feel overwhelmed and isolated.

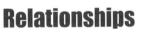 **Take a vitamin supplement**: Sustained stress levels can deplete levels of B vitamins (needed for a healthy nervous system) and magnesium, which can ease muscle tension.

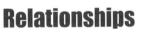 **Cut down on caffeine and alcohol**: As a stimulant, caffeine can keep you awake, and both caffeine and alcohol can contribute to anxiety and depression. Switch to decaff or herbal teas. Alcohol may make you feel sleepy initially but cause you to wake in the night, affecting the quality of your sleep.

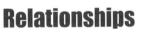 **Take regular exercise**: Even short bouts of exercise can help release 'feel-good' endorphins to boost your mood.

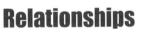 **Consider relaxation therapies**: Yoga, Tai Chi, meditation or massage which concentrate on the mind/body connection help ease stress.

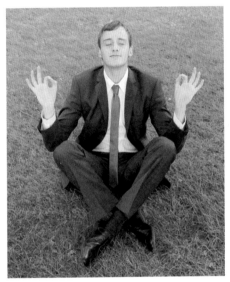

Relationships

Research has shown that people who have close relationships with partners, friends and family live longer than those who don't, so stay close. Human beings need social contact and becoming isolated can have a negative effect and result in depression and unhappiness.

Maintaining Your Relationships

Maintain your relationships by making time for them and keeping in contact. For instance, phone close family who live far away at least once a week (texts and emails just aren't the same as having a chat) and be prepared to talk through a flat mate's tough day and they will do the same for you. If your relationship with your partner hits the rocks over money, infidelity or just disillusionment with marriage, these issues all need urgent attention – counselling and marriage guidance can help.

Sleep

You'll spend a third of your life asleep. Unfortunately the demands of the 24-hour society mean most of us are actually trying to get by on less sleep – research shows that we're sleeping an hour less than our ancestors 150 years ago. Insomnia – the inability to get off to sleep or stay asleep at night is also extremely common – affecting around one in four adults. Sleep deprivation can cause daytime drowsiness, poor memory, irritability, affect relationships and work performance – so it needs to be addressed.

How Much Sleep Do You Need?

There's no text book answer to this – a lot of people quote seven to eight hours a night as the desired optimum – but the truth is it really does depend on what stage of your life you're at. Newborn babies, for instance, seem to need around 16 or 17 hours sleep a night, and children need gradually less as they get older. Despite their penchant for long lie-ins, teens only need eight to nine hours sleep a night. By your 70s you'll probably need less sleep again – around six to seven hours in some cases.

What Happens When You Sleep?

Catching up With Filing

Getting enough sleep is crucial to your physical and mental well-being. A lot of things happen while you're asleep – mainly in the brain. It's as if your body needs that time to stay on top of everything, process memories and catch up with the filing.

Producing Hormones for Maintenance

Your body produces hormones which promote the growth, repair and maintenance of muscle tissue.

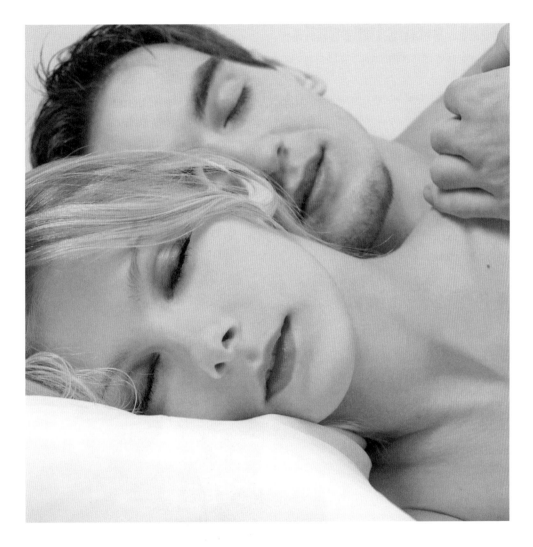

Fighting off Infections

Sleeping more can also help your body fight off infections. Experiments on mice have shown a mere seven hours of sleep deprivation can disturb the immune response – maybe one of the reasons why most of us seem more prone to infections when we've been burning the midnight oil.

What Causes Insomnia?

Disturbed sleep, problems getting to sleep or waking early have a number of causes including:

 Anxiety and stress: People who worry a lot often have sleep problems because they find it difficult to switch off. However, even if you're not a worrier it's also possible to have sleep problems during a short period of stressful circumstances such as moving house, money worries, or a bereavement.

 Caffeine, cigarettes and alcohol: Caffeine (in tea, coffee and chocolate) and cola and nicotine are all stimulants and keep you awake. All alcohol may make you feel sleepy initially; it will cause you to wake again during the night.

Depression: Disturbed sleep and early morning waking are common symptoms in people who are suffering from depression.

Medical problems: A painful medical condition such as arthritis or backache, can affect sleep and keep you awake.

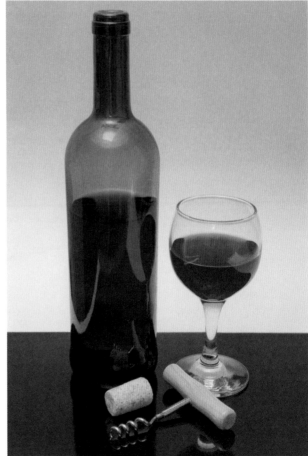

- **Disrupted routines**: Working irregular hours, especially nightshifts, can affect your body clock so it's often difficult to readjust when you need to sleep.
- **Side effects of prescription drugs**: Some medications such as statins and certain blood pressure drugs can disturb your sleep.
- **Misuse of sleeping tablets**: Most doctors only prescribe short-term doses of sleeping tablets – stopping them abruptly can also cause sleep problems.
- **Light and noise pollution**: If your curtains are too light or you live next to a busy road (or, conversely, cockerels in the countryside) you may be kept awake. Even 'too much' quiet can keep those who may be used to more ambient noise awake. Double glazing or a ticking clock, respectively, may alleviate these problems.
- **Sedentary lifestyle**: Not being active enough during the day can mean you're not tired enough to sleep.

How to Sleep Better

- **Don't panic**: Worrying about not sleeping is self-defeating and will probably make your problem worse. Most sleep problems are temporary and will resolve themselves eventually. Try keeping a sleep diary recording the pattern and quality of your sleep – you'll probably be reassured to see how much sleep you are getting.
- **Consistency**: Go to bed at the same time every night to get your body into the habit of sleeping at the same time.
- **Develop a winding down routine**: Take a warm bath, listen to some music, read and turn down the lights.
- **Spend some time in natural daylight every day**: Some research suggests working in an artificially lit office all day can cause sleep problems in office workers.
- **Cut down on caffeine**: Avoid caffeinated drinks in the evening.
- **Don't eat a heavy meal close to bedtime**: This can cause indigestion, bloating and heartburn, which will keep you awake.
- **Limit alcohol**: Although this is a depressant and can help you fall asleep, it will not

encourage quality sleep and may cause you to wake up in the middle of sleep.

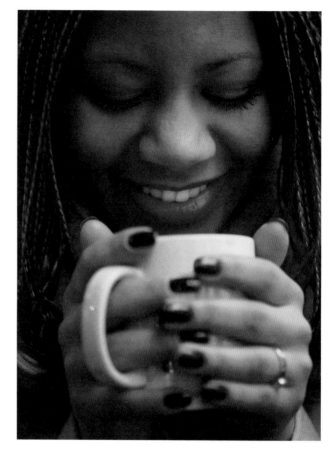

- **Avoid naps**: Don't nap for more than 20 minutes during the day, as it may reduce your chances of getting to sleep at night.
- **Exercise regularly**: Some research suggests three 20 minute exercise sessions a day helps improve the quality of your sleep, but allow three hours between exercising and bedtime to wind down.
- **Keep your bedroom cool**: Open a window a little or turn down the radiator.
- **Ban TV and laptops from the bedroom**: Your bedroom should just be for sleeping and sex.
- **Have a milky drink before bedtime**: Milk contains an amino acid called tryptophan which can induce sleepiness.
- **Sip chamomile tea**: It has a calming effect.
- **Try acupuncture**: This Chinese system of medicine which uses tiny needles to regulate the flow of energy in the body may also help.

Top Tip

Try herbal remedies such as valerian root, a remedy for insomnia since Roman times. Nutmeg has been shown to help you sleep for longer. Smelling lavender has also been shown to help.

Medical Help for Sleep Problems

If your insomnia is causing you severe distress and you have tried other non-drug options your doctor may prescribe you sleeping tablets – but only as a short-term solution. There are several types:

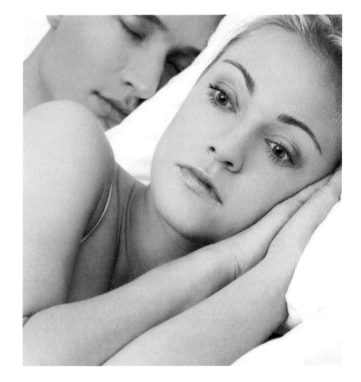

 Benzodiazepines: These are tranquillizers designed to bring down your anxiety levels. However they are potentially addictive and should only be used as a short-term solution.

 'Z' drugs: These newer type of sleeping tablet work in a similar way to benzos – but again should only be used for short-term relief of symptoms.

Melatonin: A natural hormone which governs sleep patterns, this is available in tablet form – used for short-term relief of symptoms.

Fitness and Exercise

Keeping fit by taking regular exercise is essential for maintaining a healthy lifestyle. Being active can substantially reduce your risk of dying from heart disease, helps you keep to a healthy weight and prevents disease associated with obesity. Exercise also helps improve your mood and helps you deal with stress by stimulating the production of the feel–good chemical serotonin.

How Much Exercise Do You Need?

Aim for 30 minutes brisk exercise five times a week – enough to make you a little warm and sweaty and slightly out of breath. Children need more exercise – around 60 minutes a day to help them build muscle strength, bone density and prevent them becoming overweight. However, if you're not used to exercising at this level, talk to your doctor first and get advice about how you can build up gradually.

What Type of Exercise?

You can incorporate exercise into your daily life (taking the stairs instead of the lift, walking the dog, leaving the car at home and walking the kids to school, vacuuming the house, gardening etc.) or take part in an organized exercise class or sport. Try:

- **Walking**: Brisk walking is easy to fit into your daily routine. Walking raises level of 'good' HDL cholesterol which is protective against heart disease. A 45-minute brisk walk four times a week can help you lose 18 lbs in a year. It also builds bone density (protecting against the brittle-bone disease osteoporosis) and tones up muscle. Experts recommend using a pedometer and aiming to walk 10,000 steps a day.
- **Running/Jogging**: Is one of the least expensive but most accessible ways to stay fit. It's great for cardiovascular fitness because it strengthens the heart muscle and reduces

blood pressure. It also uses more calories per minute than any other cardio exercise apart from cross-country skiing, so it's a big help in controlling weight. It is also great for stress relief.

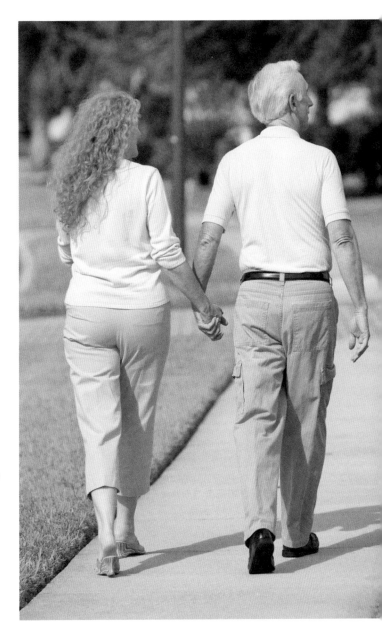

- **Dancing**: Dancing is a form of exercise most people can participate in at some level. It's great for building bone density and is beneficial for people who have heart disease, type 2 diabetes and high blood pressure. It's also very sociable.

- **Swimming**: Good 'all round' form of exercise. Swimming strengthens every muscle in the body without putting any strain on them. That's because your weight is fully supported by water. It also boosts heart and lung function, helps reduce high blood pressure, improves posture and stamina. Particularly good for overweight people, those with joint problems and pregnant women.

 Yoga: Yoga promotes both physical and mental well-being. Classes teach breathing techniques, flexibility, relaxation, better posture and sometimes meditation. It has a calming effect which is beneficial for people suffering from stress and depression.

Top Tip

Remember to warm up and warm down before and after exercising to reduce the risk of injuring yourself. Keep hydrated by drinking 300 ml to 500 ml in the 15 minutes before you work out and then about 150 ml to 250 ml every 15 minutes during exercising.

Top Tip

Try breaking your 30 minutes a day into three 10-minute segments if you're too busy – say a 10 minute walk to the train, jog around the park at lunchtime and a dog walk after work.

Checklist

- **Balance:** Eat a healthy balanced diet including five portions of fresh fruit and vegetables, lean protein, carbohydrates, fibre, calcium-rich dairy products and two portions of fish a week and go easy on saturated fats, salt and sugar.
- **Calories:** Limit your calories to no more than 1,940 for a woman and 2,550 for a man.
- **Variety:** Ensure you eat a wide range of foods to get sufficient vitamins and minerals – variety is the key.
- **Don't drink too much alcohol:** Though potentially beneficial in small amounts, any more and it is detrimental.
- **Quit smoking:** The reasons are myriad.
- **Don't take drugs:** The dangers of addiction and side effects are too great.
- **Get enough sleep:** You'll be able to work out how much you need from how you feel in the mornings.
- **Manage your stress levels:** Learn to relax and switch off.
- **Take plenty of exercise:** Aim for five 30-minute sessions a week.
- **Stay close to friends and family:** It's crucial for your mental health.

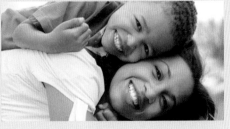

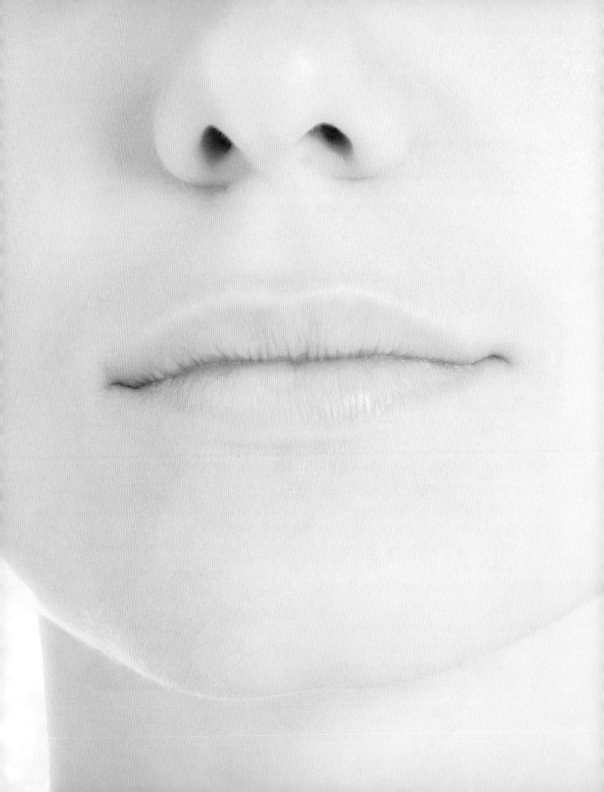

Head & Neck Health

The Brain and Nervous System

Your brain is arguably the most important organ in your body. It is the command centre that controls all bodily functions including digestion, breathing, heart rate, blood pressure and coordination of movement. It is also responsible for consciousness, allowing you to think, store memories, learn and create. The brain regulates and coordinates all these functions supported by nerve impulses that travel up and down the spinal cord.

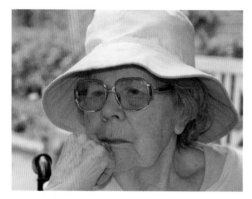

Dementia

Dementia is a group of related symptoms associated with a degeneration of the brain and the way it functions. It affects one in 14 people over the age of 65 and one in six people over the age of 80. Although it mainly affects the elderly, certain types of dementia can also affect younger people. The two most common kinds are described below.

Alzheimer's Disease

This is the most common type of dementia and is associated with plaques of an abnormal protein deposited in brain tissue. No-one knows what causes Alzheimer's for sure but it's likely to be a combination of age, genetics and environmental factors. Boxers and other people who have suffered severe head injuries are at higher risk of Alzheimer's disease, as are people who smoke, or have high blood pressure and/or raised cholesterol. Symptoms get worse as the disease progresses and include:

 Memory lapses and difficulty finding the correct word
Confusion and increasingly losing the ability to plan

Mood swings; anger, sadness, fear and/or frustration at the loss of memory

Withdrawal due to loss of confidence or communication problems

There are a number of tests that can be performed in order to diagnose Alzheimer's:

 Detailed psychological tests such as memory and cognitive function tests

Blood tests, done to eliminate vascular dementia (*see* page 58)

Brain scans such as a CT or MRI scan will be able to detect changes taking place in the brain

Treatment for Alzheimer's can include:

 Drugs: Drugs can boost levels of a chemical called acetylcholine in the brain. The best-known one is called Aricept (donepezil hydrochloride) and is suitable if you have moderate disease. It doesn't cure Alzheimer's but it can stabilize symptoms. Another drug called Ebixa (memantine) is for patients in the mid–late stages of Alzheimer's and acts by preventing excess calcium ions entering into brain cells. In cases where the patient is aggressive or agitated, anti-psychotic drugs can be prescribed. However these should be reserved for the most severe cases because they increase the risk of stroke. Be aware that sometimes the side effects from medications can outweigh benefits.

Psychological treatment: Strategies which may help include exercises and problem-solving tasks designed to improve your memory, such as crosswords.

Exercise therapy: This can improve mobility as well as boost mood and mental function.

Personal care package: This can help to maintain the dignity of the patient, either at home or in a nursing home.

Top Tip

Jog your memory by keeping a diary, writing dates on a calendar, keeping your keys in an obvious place and using picture–association to try and remember names.

Vascular Dementia

This type of dementia is caused by an interruption of blood supply to the brain, which causes brain cells to become damaged and die. It can happen as a result of a stroke (where a clot blocks an artery in the brain) or less severe blockages called mini-strokes. It can also be caused by tiny blood vessels in the brain narrowing and hardening. Some of the symptoms are the same as for Alzheimer's, such as memory loss, difficulties with concentration and planning. They also include:

 Stroke-like symptoms (such as muscle weakness and partial paralysis – *see* Stroke, page 133)

Change in personality and mood

Walking slowly and unsteadily

Depression

Treatments for vascular dementia concentrate on slowing down existing health conditions such as stroke, high blood pressure and raised cholesterol. They include:

 Medication to lower blood pressure and cholesterol

Lifestyle changes such as quitting smoking, cutting down on alcohol and eating a healthy diet

Rehabilitation help such as speech therapy and physiotherapy

Antidepressants may be prescribed if symptoms are depression

Sleeping tablets such as the 'Z' group of drugs (*see* insomnia page 46) may be prescribed if sleep is disturbed

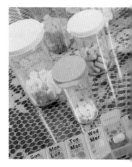

Epilepsy

Epilepsy is the name for recurrent seizures caused by a sudden burst of excess electrical activity in the brain. There are various different types of epilepsy and seizures will vary in their severity and frequency. Epilepsy isn't usually considered life threatening in itself; it's just that you may injure yourself while you are having a seizure. However, in rare cases there are sudden deaths from epilepsy that cannot be explained by a post-mortem.

What Causes it and Who Gets it?

Sometimes epilepsy can begin after a brain injury caused by a blow to the head or meningitis, but in most cases there is no obvious cause. It can start at any stage in life but usually begins in childhood. One in 20 people will have a seizure at some point in their life, and around one in 130 people will have recurrent seizures. One in 280 children is affected and it's more common in people with a learning disability.

Symptoms

These vary but can include:
- A trance-like state
- Loss of consciousness
- Uncontrollable shaking of the body

Did You Know?

Forty per cent of children and 30 per cent of adults are wrongly diagnosed with epilepsy. In many cases their 'seizures' are actually blackouts caused by an irregular heartbeat. Misdiagnosis could be avoided by patients having a 12-lead ECG measurement.

Diagnosis and Treatment

You should see an epilepsy specialist in order to be diagnosed. He will use an electro-encephalogram to record your brain wave activity and listen to your description of your seizures before making a diagnosis. The good news is that 70 per cent of patients are able to control their disease with medication. These drugs are known as anti-epileptic drugs. The drug you are prescribed will depend on the type of epilepsy you have. You must report your seizures to driving authorities. If they are uncontrolled you may have to give up your driver's licence.

Migraine

Migraine is one of the most common neurological conditions; a type of headache with quite distinctive symptoms (see below). The headaches can last several days and be very debilitating. Migraine attacks are much more common amongst women than men.

Symptoms

A migraine can start out of the blue or build up with a series of pre-attack warnings signs such as tiredness, yawning, hyperactivity, mood swings and food cravings. Symptoms vary but can include:

 Throbbing pain, usually on one side of the head

Visual disturbances, such as flashing lights or blind spots

Nausea and/or vomiting

Increased sensitivity to sounds, lights and smells

Stiff neck and shoulders

Neurological symptoms or 'aura', such as tingling in the limbs and concentration problems (affecting about one in 10 migraine sufferers)

Prevention

Migraine has a number of known triggers connected with the release of a chemical from the brain called serotonin into the bloodstream. If you're having frequent and severe attacks your doctor may prescribe drugs to prevent migraines such as the anti-depressant amitriptyline or beta blockers. Try avoiding these known triggers (where possible!) to avoid attacks:

Stress and emotional issues

Tiredness or changes in routine and sleeping pattern

Foods such as chocolate, cheese, citrus fruits and red wine

Dehydration or fasting

Bright or flickering lights

Loud high-pitched noise

Hormones (PMS, puberty, menopause)

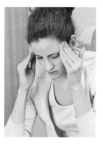

Treatment

There are a number of strategies which may help relieve your symptoms, such as resting in a quiet dark room, applying a hot or cold compress and taking a fast-acting soluble painkiller (for mild to moderate pain) as soon as you feel the symptoms coming on. Other drugs include:

- **Triptan drugs**: These stop the effects of serotonin. One example is sumatriptan. They are available as sprays, tablets, injections, nasal sprays or dissolvable wafers.
- **Anti-sickness drugs**: These drugs can also help ease nausea. Examples include metoclopramide and domperidone.

Did You Know?

Sometimes painkillers don't work because they are not absorbed, as the stomach has 'gone on strike'. The anti-sickness drugs mentioned here help to move the stomach contents on so that the pain relief drugs can be taken into the body.

Parkinson's Disease

This is a neurological disease which affects the way the brain coordinates body movements, including walking and talking. It affects all ages, but is more common in the over 50s. It is caused by loss of nerve cells in the part of your brain responsible for producing a chemical called dopamine, which transmits messages from your brain to coordinate movements.

Symptoms

There are three main symptoms:

- **Tremor (shaking), usually in one hand or arm, and is more likely when resting**
- **Stiff, tense, rigid muscles**
- **Slowness of movement – simple tasks like getting out of bed may take longer**

Treatment

- **Drugs**: At the moment there is no cure for Parkinson's disease but a number of drug treatments can help control symptoms; these include Levodopa which is absorbed by the nerve cells in the brain and turned into dopamine (an important chemical involved in movement control). Your doctor may also want to try newer drugs as well.
- **Surgery**: Chronic brain stimulation involves implanting a pacemaker-like device into your chest wall where it generates an electrical current to stimulate part of your brain affected by Parkinson's disease.

Mental health and Wellbeing

A well-balanced personality is crucial to good health. Around one in four people suffer from mental health problems at some point in their life, ranging from depression through to eating disorders, bipolar disorder and schizophrenia.

Depression

Around 15 per cent of people with depression suffer a severe episode during their lifetime. If you're depressed you'll experience feelings of profound sadness for weeks or months, and those feelings may affect your relationships, social life, self-esteem and performance at work.

Symptoms

These can include both psychological, social and physical symptoms including:

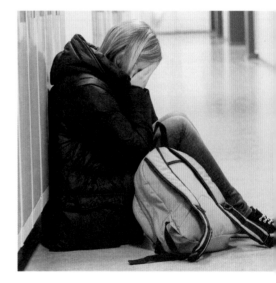

- Feelings of sadness
- Low self esteem
- Tearfulness
- Anxiety/worrying
- Difficulties in making any decisions
- Lack of enjoyment
- Low libido
- Changes in appetite
- Reduced energy levels
- Disturbed sleep patterns particularly early morning waking
- Poor performance at work
- Avoiding social contact
- Family/relationship problems

Diagnosis and Treatment

There's no diagnostic test for depression. Your doctor will make a diagnosis based on your description of your symptoms. Treatment options include antidepressants and psychological therapies, plus some herbal remedies.

 Drug treatments: These include a type of antidepressants called selective serotonin reuptake inhibitors (SSRIs) which work by increasing levels of the 'feel-good' brain chemical serotonin. They can take up to four weeks to have an effect on your mood. Other antidepressants which work in different ways are also prescribed.

Psychological therapies: These include counselling and cognitive behavioural therapy (CBT – a talking therapy which can help you challenge negative thought patterns).

Herbal remedies: St John's Wort is a natural antidepressant, but cannot be taken if you are taking certain medications, including the contraceptive pill and antidepressants. Before taking this preparaton seek advice from your pharmacist or doctor.

Did You Know?

Clinical studies have shown that a diet rich in omega-3 fatty acids may help protect against depression.

Manic Depression (Bipolar Disorder)

This is a type of depression which involves extreme mood swings, alternating between deep depression to periods of overactive, excited or 'manic' behaviour. It affects up to two per cent of the population. Stress seems to be the most significant trigger, and bipolar disorder can run in families. Many cases, however, have no obvious genetic factor involved.

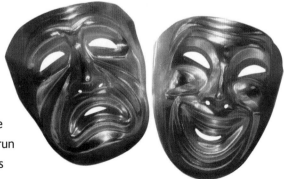

Depression symptoms: These include feelings of despair, guilt and worthlessness, weight gain, sleeping difficulties, concentration problems and sometimes suicidal feelings.

 Mania symptoms: These can include feelings of euphoria, a heightened sense of self-importance, extravagant spending, ambitious schemes, increased libido and also anger and irritability.

Treatment

 Drugs: Lithium is often prescribed for bipolar disorder. Side effects can include dry mouth, weight gain and tremor, but it is usually well tolerated – your doctor will want you to have regular blood tests to monitor lithium blood levels and check on other systems. Other drugs prescribed include anti-convulsants to stabilize mood.

 Talking therapies: Counselling and psychotherapy can help you understand your feelings and change the way you think and feel.

 Hospital stay: Treatment as an in-patient can give you a chance to rest and be assessed to work out the most effective treatments for you.

Schizophrenia

Schizophrenia is a type of mental illness known as 'psychosis', where the patient loses touch with reality. Most people with schizophrenia are diagnosed between the ages of 15 and 35. The condition affects one in 100 people. Symptoms can include:

 Strange illogical thinking: People with schizophrenia may be unable to follow logical thought processes and find conversation difficult.

 Hallucinations and delusions: These can include hearing voices that others don't hear, mostly critical or unfriendly, or believing that other people can control them or read their minds.

Becoming withdrawn, apathetic or unable to concentrate: This can lead to feelings of loneliness and isolation and a further sense of unreality.

Causes

Experts believe a number of factors may be associated with schizophrenia. These include:

 Genetic predisposition: Experts don't believe there is a schizophrenia gene but it may be that a combination of genes may make you more likely to develop schizophrenia.

Stressful life events: Being jobless, homeless, suffering bereavement or being the victim of physical or sexual abuse or other life-changing events may trigger schizophrenia.

Smoking cannabis: This has been associated with schizophrenia (*see* page 38).

Treatment

Drug treatments: These include antipsychotic drugs, which have a sedative effect and can help to make the 'voices' more tolerable and less intrusive, but if you are prescribed these you will need close monitoring because of the risk of side effects.

 Psychological treatments: These include counselling, psychotherapy and CBT (*see* page 63).

Eating Disorders

Food can become a problem if you use it to cope with emotions such as boredom, anxiety, stress, sadness, loneliness or anger. An eating disorder is characterized by an abnormal attitude to food including controlling how much is eaten. Eating disorders can affect *anyone from any age group or sex*, but are most common in young women aged 15–25, although 10 per cent of cases occur in men and they can also appear for the first time in middle age.

Causes

It's likely that a combination of factors can trigger eating disorders. Stressful events such as being bullied, sexual abuse, divorce, bereavement or mental health problems such as lack of confidence, low self esteem and loneliness can all act as triggers. There are two main types of eating disorder (*see* below).

Anorexia Nervosa

People with anorexia restrict the amount they eat and drink to a dangerously low level as a way of demonstrating control over their body weight. Chemical changes in the brain eventually distort their thinking so that they can't take rational decisions about food and suffer malnutrition and exhaustion. Some anorexics literally starve themselves to death. Symptoms include:

- **Dangerous restriction of food and drink**
- **Extreme weight loss**
- **Dizzy spells and/or fainting**
- **Cessation of periods (can develop infertility in long term)**
- **Constipation and/or stomach pains**
- **Bloated stomach**

- Dry skin
- Downy hair appearing on the body
- Intense fear of gaining weight
- Distorted view of body shape
- Personality changes and mood swings
- Feeling cold

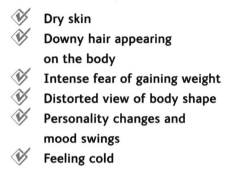

Did You Know?

Eating disorders are common amongst young women with families who don't communicate well, but have high expectations, and also among gay men.

A range of psychological therapies and self-help strategies including counselling, family therapy, group therapy, drama or arts therapy, nutrition and advice from eating disorder support groups, can help combat anorexia, but the sufferer will need expert help and careful physical monitoring.

Bulimia

A person with bulimia has an uncontrollable urge to eat huge amounts of foods – in an attempt to fill an emotional hunger that can't be satisfied – and then use vomiting and/or laxatives or diuretics as a means of controlling their weight. People with bulimia can be harder to identify than those with anorexia because they frequently are in the normal weight range and their bingeing/vomiting takes place in private. Telltale signs include:

- Mood swings
- Abrasions on the back of their hands, caused by their teeth grazing the hand they stick down their throat to induce vomiting
- Frequent sore throats
- Tooth decay, due to acid from vomit attacking their tooth enamel

Psychological therapies can help; particularly cognitive behavioural therapies (see page 63) which can help you get a more positive attitude to food and eating.

Hair and Scalp

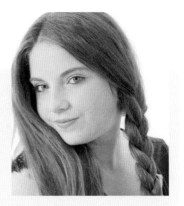

Hair loss can be a very distressing condition, particularly for women. Hair loss in men is more socially acceptable (*see* male pattern baldness, page 154). Scalp health can be very important for the appearance of the hair and a flaky scalp can cause unsightly and embarrassing dandruff.

Hair Loss

All of us lose about 150 hairs a day normally, and it often occurs as a temporary natural phenomenon after childbirth. However, the medical name for *significant* hair loss from the scalp or beard (and less frequently the eyelashes and eyebrows) is alopecia areata. It's quite common and affects around 15 in 10,000 people.

Causes and Symptoms

Alopecia areata is an auto-immune disease, the body starts attacking its own hair follicles. In one in four cases there is a family history of the disease. Stress is also thought to be a factor, and it is worth checking blood tests for anaemia and thyroid functioning. Symptoms are:

- Round, smooth bald patches appear on the scalp or within beards
- Short broken hairs, which may appear around the edges
- Sudden onset – hair loss usually starts abruptly

Treatment

The good news is that most mild hair loss will regrow, so your doctor will probably advise a 'watch and wait' policy. However, if you have more than 50 per cent hair loss and there is no sign of any regrowth, you may be referred to a dermatologist. Treatment options include:

Topical corticosteroids: These have immunosuppressant effects and include lotions, gel and foam, creams and ointments. They'll usually be prescribed for three months initially.

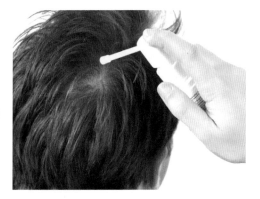

 Topical immunotherapy: This causes an allergic contact dermatitis, which can stimulate hair regrowth. It involves multiple hospital or clinic visits and has only a 50 per cent success rate.

 Wigs: Made of either acrylic or real hair, wigs can help conceal hair loss.

Counselling: Losing your hair can be extremely distressing and talking therapies can help you come to terms with your loss.

Did You Know?

Research has shown that 80 per cent of people with less than 40 per cent hair loss can expect regrowth within a year, even without treatment.

Other types of alopecia

There are many different kinds of alopecia. Here is a guide to some of the most common types.

Androgenic alopecia: Also known as male pattern baldness (*see* page 154). Female androgenic alopecia usually involves thinning hair over the crown.

Alopecia totalis: This is the medical name for total hair loss on the scalp and can happen around three months after a significant event such as physical or psychological stress. It usually lasts 3 to 6 months and in most cases will grow back.

Tinea capitis: A fungal scalp infection which mostly affects children. It causes patchy hair loss and may itch and appear scaly.

Excess Hair

Excess hair (hirsutism) is a fairly common complaint amongst women, especially above the upper lip. There are several measures that can be undertaken, including medication in the form of a special cream. However, hirsutism can be a symptom of a whole range of conditions from polycystic ovary syndrome to insulin resistance, so talk to your doctor if at all concerned.

Dandruff

Dandruff is characterized by flaky white skin appearing on the scalp and can vary in severity – proving more socially embarrassing than a medical problem. Babies sometimes develop it too (known as cradle cap).

Causes

Skin cells are shed naturally from your scalp every day; if more than the normal number are lost they can clump together and form dandruff. It's more common where the skin on the scalp is either too oily (such as during puberty) or too dry. Sometimes the scalp can become inflamed.

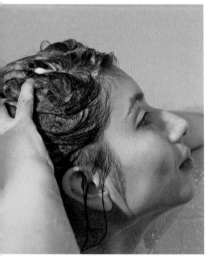

Treatment

- **Shampoos**: These are specially formulated to tackle dandruff and fungus and are available to buy from pharmacies. Look for active ingredients including zinc pyrithione, coal tar, selenium sulphide, salicyclic acids and Ketoconazole.
- **Steroid scalp applications**: These are sometimes prescribed for severe cases.
- **Regular hair brushing**: This can prevent build-up of dead skin cells.
- **Flaxseed oil (linseed)**: This may help dandruff too; try a teaspoonful in your daily diet.

Eyes

Eyesight is one of our most important senses, although many of us neglect day-to-day maintenance. It's important to have an eye test at least once every two years and once a year if you are aged over 60.

Eye Diseases

Optometrists, and most opticians, are trained to spot early signs of eye diseases, which include:

Glaucoma

This is when the pressure of the fluid in the eye is so high that it causes damage. If any close relatives have a history of glaucoma, speak to your optician about regular eye pressure checks.

Diabetic Retinopathy

A complication of diabetes where the retina (the light-sensitive area at the back of the eye) and the blood vessels serving it become damaged.

Macular Degeneration

This affects the macula, part of the retina which is responsible for fine detail at the centre of field of vision and results in loss of detailed central vision – faces are unclear, for example.

Cataracts

These occur when the eye lens becomes cloudy and vision less clear and detailed. Cataracts mainly affect elderly people.

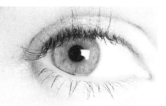

Colour Blindness

This is caused by a defect in cone cells at the back of the retina which interpret colour. Types of colour blindness include red/green colour blindness, which is the inability to distinguish between certain shades of these two colours, blue/yellow blindness, where yellow can appear as purple, and total colour blindness, where everything is seen in shades of black, white and grey. Colour blindness affects one in 20 men and one in 200 women and is mainly an inherited condition (although it can also develop as a side effect of medication or a pre-existing medical condition). It can be difficult to detect; you may be unaware that what you are seeing is not the right colour. However optometrists can detect red/green colour blindness using the Ishihara test, which tests coloured visions using coloured plates.

Treatment

No treatment is currently available for inherited colour blindness. Pilots or coastguards require good colour vision so they are not suitable jobs for you if you are colour blind. For acquired colour blindness, once the underlying cause has been identified and treated, your coloured vision may return.

Conjunctivitis

This is the name for an irritation or inflammation of the conjunctiva, a transparent layer of cells that covers the eye. There are three types: irritant (caused by an irritant in your eye, such as grit or an eyelash), allergic (an allergen gets into the eye, such as pollen or pet hair), and infective (caused by bacteria, a virus or a sexually transmitted disease). Symptoms are:

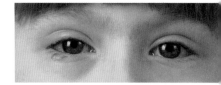

- Reddening of the eye
- Watering of the eye
- Sticky discharge which clogs up the eyelashes

Treatment

Most cases of conjunctivitis resolve on their own within seven days. Some doctors prescribe antibiotic creams if an attack fails to clear up. Antihistamines can also be used to dampen down allergic conjunctivitis. You can speed up the healing process by: frequent hand washing, using lubricant eye drops, removing any discharge, and taking out your contact lenses.

Ears

Your ear is the organ responsible for hearing and balance. Ear infections and other conditions such as blockages due to ear wax and tinnitus (a sensation that noise is coming from within the body rather than outside) are extremely common. Hearing loss becomes more common with age due to damage to the hair cells within the cochlea or as a side effect of some cancer drugs, rubella or a head injury.

Ear-wax Blockages

Ear wax is a combination of sebum, dead skin cells and a wax-like substance, which cleans, lubricates and protects the lining of the ear by trapping dirt and repelling water. It also has antibacterial and antifungal properties. A build-up of excessive ear wax can cause:

 Earache   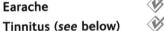 Temporary hearing loss

Tinnitus (*see below*)   Vertigo (a spinning sensation when standing still)

Treatment

Many cases resolve on their own, without the need for treatment, but ear drops and ear irrigation can also help. Ear drops are made up of olive or almond oil, sodium chloride and sodium bicarbonate and help by softening earwax, while ear irrigation involves cleaning out the ears with a pressurised jet of water to remove build-up.

Earache and Ear Infections

Pain in the ear is extremely common, especially amongst children (75 per cent of cases are in children under 10). The most frequent cause is infection of the middle ear, caused by bacteria or a virus and a build-up fluid/pus, resulting in discomfort and pain. Symptoms can include:

Earache

 Temporary hearing loss

 High temperature

 Blood and pus oozing from the ear

Treatment

Most middle-ear infections get better on their own within three days, but paracetamol or ibuprofen can help relieve pain and bring down fever. If the pain hasn't gone after three days your doctor may prescribe antibiotics. (*See also* Glue ear, page 201).

Otitis Externa

This is an inflammation of the outer ear canal. Its causes include infection, allergy or water in the ear, resulting in itching, pain, dulled hearing and/or discharge. Treatment includes antibiotic and steroidal ear drops, and painkillers.

Tinnitus

This is a ringing, buzzing or whistling sound or other noise that you perceive to be coming from inside the ear or your head, rather than outside. It is an extremely common hearing condition and is said to affect around one third of adults to some degree; only about one in 100 will suffer long-term problems though. Tinnitus is frequently associated with hearing loss due to exposure to loud noise (such as a rock concert) and continuous exposure to a noisy environment (such as a factory or aircraft hangar). It can also be connected with other ear diseases, such as otitis media.

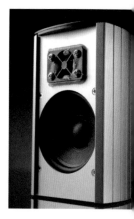

Treatment

There's no cure for tinnitus but treatments can help sufferers cope with the disease. These include:

 White noise generators, which emit a low-level background noise to distract from the tinnitus

 Background noise such as radio or TV

 Listening to music

 Relaxation therapies

 Counselling

The Nose

The nose contains the upper region of the respiratory tract and is involved in breathing and is also responsible for smell. A number of medical problems affect the nose including the common cold, hay fever and other allergies, blocked sinus passages, nosebleeds and snoring.

The Common Cold

There are more than 200 different cold viruses and most of us will catch at least two colds a year. We get more colds in winter because we spend more time indoors in close contact with others. The cold virus is spread by tiny droplets being sneezed or coughed out. In most cases a cold will clear up within seven days, without the need for any treatment. The symptoms include a blocked up or runny nose, sneezing, a sore throat, and/or a cough.

Treatment

There's still no cure for the common cold, but you can relieve your symptoms by:

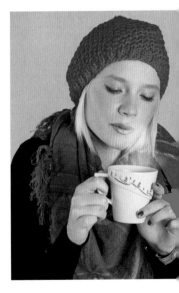

- Drinking lots of hot fluids
- Resting as much as possible
- Taking paracetamol- or ibuprofen-based cold remedies
- Eating a healthy diet (*see* pages 18–33)
- Using nasal decongestants to 'unblock' a snuffly nose
- Breathing in steam from a bowl of boiling water with a towel over your head, to loosen mucus
- Popular natural remedies for colds include Echinacea, black elderberry extract, high doses of vitamin C and zinc – despite little evidence to show they work

Complications

If your symptoms don't seem to be improving you should see your doctor as it's possible you could have developed a bacterial infection in the chest or sinuses and may need antibiotics.

Catarrh

Catarrh is the name given to a build-up of mucus in the nasal cavities, often occurring as a complication of a cold. It may also affect the throat, ears and chest. It causes congestion and the coughing-up of green phlegm. Oral or nasal decongestants should help relieve the problem and clear it up after a few days; antihistamines may help if you develop a long-term chronic problem caused by an allergy; and steam inhalation may also help (*see* page 75).

Sinusitis

This can develop as a complication of the common cold and is caused by congestion (a build-up of mucus) in the sinus passages – air-filled spaces in the bones of the skull that open in the nose. Symptoms include: pain over the cheeks, forehead or bridge of nose, a blocked nose and green catarrh (*see* above). Treatment can include antibiotics, decongestants (such as xylometazoline) – though long-term use of these can exacerbate the congestion, and possibly surgical drainage for long-term sufferers, which involves irrigating the nose with saline (salt water). However, there is currently research being undertaken to ascertain whether drainage can be medically proven to work.

Seasonal Flu

Between five and 20 per cent of us will get a dose of flu every year. Like the common cold, flu is a respiratory illness and can sometimes be difficult to distinguish from a cold (*see* below). This is because some of the symptoms are the same, such as sore throat, cough and blocked and runny nose. In most cases you'll feel better after five to seven days unless you develop a complication (*see* above).

Is it Flu or a Cold?

Flu symptoms are usually more serious than those of a cold, and accompanied by:

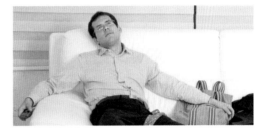

- Feelings of extreme fatigue
- Sudden fever of 38°C (100.4°F)
- Aching muscles and joint or limb pain
- Headache
- Stomach upsets (especially in children)

Treatment

Prevention is better than cure, so if you are eligible for a flu jab, get one. They have been shown to be very effective at preventing or reducing the effects of flu. Relieve flu symptoms by:

- **Taking paracetamol or similar analgesics**: Most cases of flu get better on their own and you can relieve symptoms in the same way as for the common cold (see page 75).

- **Anti-viral drugs**: If you're are in a high risk health group (aged over 65, diabetic, have impaired immunity or suffering from chronic lung disease, heart disease, kidney disease or a neurological disease like Parkinson's or MS) you may need to see your doctor within the first 48 hours of your symptoms beginning for anti-viral drugs such as zanamivir (Relenza) or oseltamivir (Tamiflu).
- **Antibiotics**: These can be prescribed for bacterial infections that develop as a complication.

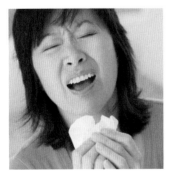

Hay Fever

Hay fever is a form of allergic rhinitis caused by the body mounting an allergic response to pollen. The body makes an allergic antibody called IgE and this triggers the release of chemicals in the nose, eyes or airways which cause inflammation and irritation, resulting in sneezing, a runny nose, streaming eyes and/or itchy eyes.

Treatment

✅ **Avoid triggers**: Easier said than done but try to follow common sense tips like checking pollen counts daily in the spring/summer months, wearing wraparound sunglasses and keeping the house and car windows shut.

✅ **Use antihistamines**: These work on a chemical called histamine, which is released by the body as part of an allergic response. They include tablets and nasal sprays. Try several brands, and remember that some can have sedative effects – read the label.

✅ **Steroid nasal spray**: If antihistamines fail to control your symptoms, these may be more effective.

✅ **Desensitization/Immunotherapy**: This involves a course of injections and sometimes tablets containing minute quantities of the type of pollen you are allergic to, but is usually reserved for the most serious cases as it is very time-consuming to administer.

Snoring

About one in four people are regular snorers. It's a noise caused by the soft palate (at the back of the roof of your mouth) and other tissue in the mouth, throat and nose, vibrating when air does not flow smoothly through air passages.

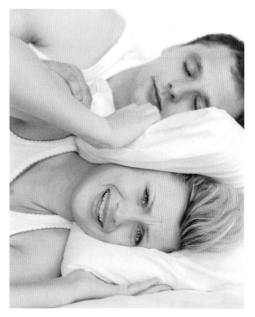

Causes

The airways can be obstructed by a number of factors including:

✅ **Being older**: The muscles at the back of your throat are weaker and more likely to vibrate.

Alcohol: Can relax the muscles at the back of your throat, palate etc. making them more likely to vibrate.

 Sleeping position: If you sleep on your back you are more likely to snore.

Smoking: Smoke can irritate the lining of your nose and throat causing swelling, which obstructs the airways.

Weight: *See 'Did You Know?'*

Sleep apnoea: Snoring may also be a sign of a condition called sleep apnoea where obstruction of your airways stops you breathing for a few seconds, waking you up at night and making you feel tired the next day.

Treatment

✔ Self–help measures such as losing weight, not drinking alcohol within four hours of bedtime, quitting smoking and sleeping on your side

✔ Antihistamine drugs to clear nasal congestion

✔ Eucalyptus oil sprinkled on your pillowcase to clear your airways

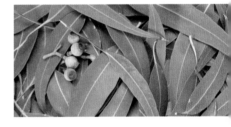

✔ Adhesive nasal strips/chin strips to encourage you to breathe through your nose

✔ Other products designed to combat snoring (see the websites section at the back of this book)

✔ Nose or throat surgery – your doctor may be able to refer you for this if the above don't work and your symptoms are severe

Did You Know?

If you're overweight, extra fat around your neck can cause sagging of tissues and obstruct air flow. If you have a collar size of 17 inches or over you may not have the muscle tone to keep your airways open.

Mouth

The mouth is the first stage in the digestion of food. It is also used for breathing and as part of the speech process. Good oral hygiene is vitally important for healthy teeth and gums and fresh breath.

Bad Breath

If you suspect you have bad breath; lick the inside of your wrist and then sniff it – if it's a bit whiffy you probably have smelly breath too. You may also notice that you have an unpleasant taste in your mouth.

Causes

- **Poor dental hygiene**: Bacteria that coat your teeth and gums can give off smelly gases if they are not removed by regular brushing and flossing. Brushing removes only 60 per cent of the plaque on your teeth.
- **Dry mouth**: If you have insufficient saliva flow you may notice a dry mouth and bad breath. This can be a side effect of certain types of medication.
- **Gum disease**: *see* page 81.
- **Strong-smelling foods**: Onions, garlic and coffee can all cause temporary bad breath.
- **Symptom of another infection**: These include bacteria infections like bronchitis and sinusitis.

Prevention and Treatment

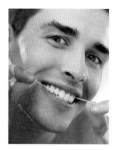

- **Regular brushing twice a day with fluoride toothpaste**
- **Cleaning by a dental hygienist**
- **Flossing and interdental brushing**

Tongue brushing

 Mouthwash specially formulated for gum disease

Top Tip

Chewing sugar-free gum can prevent bad breath by stimulating saliva flow.

Bleeding Gums and Gum Disease

If your gums bleed when you brush them and are red and swollen instead of pink then you may have gum disease, a common cause of tooth loss. All gum disease is caused by build-up of plaque – a film of bacteria that forms on your teeth and gums.

Types of Gum Disease

There are two stages of gum disease: gingivitis, which is an inflammation of the gums, and periodontal disease, which occurs when long-standing inflammation begins to affect the tissue supporting the tooth and if left untreated can lead to bone loss in the jaw eventually resulting in tooth loss.

Prevention and Treatment

See the good oral hygiene tips above. If you develop periodontal disease your dentist may have to clean the roots of your tooth, a procedure called root planning.

Cold Sores

These are small blisters on the corner of the mouth caused by the herpes simplex virus and can feel painful and look unsightly. They usually last five to seven days. You may notice a tingling feeling when one is about to appear. They can also appear on the hands and genitals and are highly infectious so avoid touching them. Once you've been infected with the virus it can reoccur at any time. Treatments

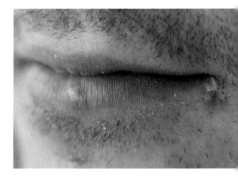

include the use of an anti-viral cream, such as acyclovir, to soothe pain and speed up healing, and wearing a sunblock if you find sunlight triggers an outbreak.

Mouth Ulcers

Around one in five people experience recurrent mouth ulcers. They can be small (between two and eight mm) or large. They are round or oval and white, grey or yellow in colour. They can also look inflamed (red). They tend to appear on the inside of the mouth or under the tongue.

Causes

Possible triggers can include stress, iron and vitamin B12 deficiencies, hormone changes (such as around the time of a period), side effects of certain drugs, and certain foods, including wheat flour, tomatoes, peanuts, almonds, strawberries and chocolate.

Prevention and Treatment

Mouth ulcers can be prevented by:

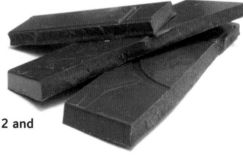

 Avoiding triggers (listed above)
Using a soft bristle toothbrush
Getting tested and treated for vitamin B12 and iron deficiency (*see* pages 23 and 25)

Treatment options include:

 Topical and drug treatments: Try using specially formulated pain-killing gels, mouthwashes or corticosteroids. Alternatively, try putting salt onto your damp little finger and apply it directly onto the ulcer for a few minutes, three times a day, then rinse your mouth out with tap water. Beware, it will make you dribble and, yes, it does sting!

Get a check-up: Severe mouth ulcers that persist for more than three weeks need investigation as in rare cases they could be a sign of mouth cancer.

The Neck

The neck is an important region of the body housing powerful muscles to support the head and control the jaw, as well as the larynx, the windpipe (trachea) and oesophagus, plus major blood vessels leading to the head.

Laryngitis

Laryngitis is an inflammation of the larynx (voice box). It is usually caused by a virus and can be associated with a common cold infection. Symptoms include:

- **Hoarse throat; sometimes your voice is lost completely or reduced to a croak**
- **Sore throat**
- **Raised temperature**
- **Repeated need to clear throat**
- **Cough**

Treatment

Acute laryngitis usually goes away on its own; as it's caused by a virus, antibiotics are not prescribed. A hoarse voice that doesn't resolve after three weeks is known as chronic laryngitis and it needs investigation to rule out other more serious causes. The following tips may help relieve symptoms of acute laryngitis:

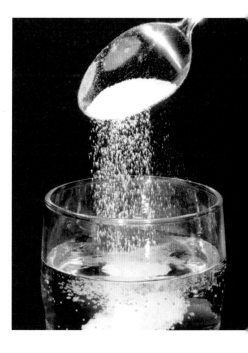

- **Rest your voice**
- **Keep hydrated**
- **Gargle with salt water**
- **Take painkillers (ibuprofen or paracetamol)**

Strep A Throat

Strep throat infection is the name for symptoms associated with Group A streptococcus bacteria and accounts for approximately 10 per cent of all sore throats. Symptoms include:

- Severe sore throat – with visible redness
- High temperature which develops quickly
- Tonsil inflammation
- Swollen lymph nodes in the neck
- Headache

Top Tip

If your sore throat doesn't disappear or you develop a rash, you should seek medical attention. Always be aware that it might be glandular fever, especially if the sufferer is a teenager.

Treatment

Your doctor can diagnose strep throat using a swab test and antibiotics may be prescribed to prevent complications developing, such as scarlet fever (a distinctive rash accompanied by sore throat and fever, caused by Streptococcus pyogenes).

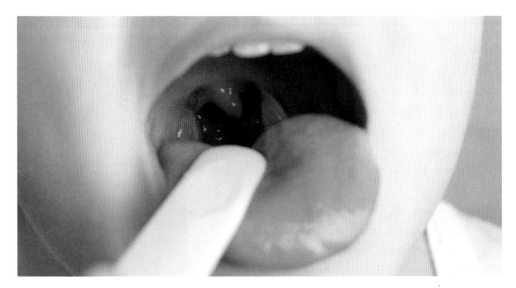

Tonsillitis

This is an infection of the tonsils (small glands at the back of the throat, which are believed to help protect against upper respiratory tract infections). It can be caused by a virus or a bacterial infection. Tonsillitis is very common in children and can become a recurring problem. Symptoms include:

- **Sore throat**
- **Fever**
- **Earache**
- **Visibly inflamed tonsils, sometimes with white spots**
- **Headache**
- **Swollen lymph nodes in the neck**

Treatment

Treatment options include painkillers such as ibuprofen and paracetamol, antibiotics for bacterial tonsillitis (although they don't alter the duration of the illness much) and surgery – an operation to remove the tonsils is considered if a child has five or more recurrent attacks, but this operation is performed less these days as it has been shown to have little long-term benefit.

Checklist

- **Watch your memory**: Get any memory problems checked out as early as possible.
- **Avoid known triggers for migraine**: These include stress, cheese, chocolate, red wine, high-pitched loud noises and flashing lights.
- **Get support if you have depression symptoms**: If you feel sad, tearful, anxious or have low self esteem – antidepressants and talking therapies can help.
- **Have your eyes checked**: Have an eye test at least once every two years and once a year if you are aged over 60.
- **Practise good oral hygiene**: Brush twice a day with a fluoride toothpaste and floss to remove plaque.

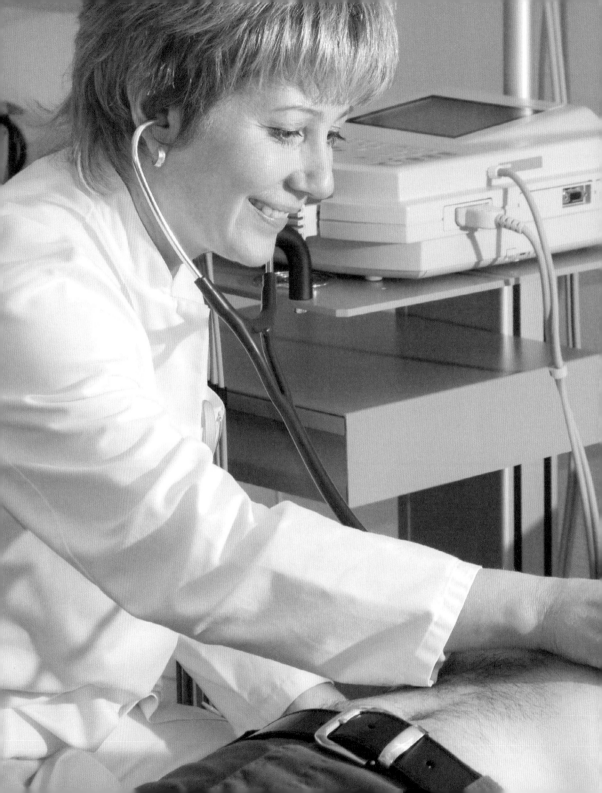

Chest & Abdominal Health

Chest, Heart and Lungs

Your chest contains some of the most important organs in your body: the heart and lungs. The health of these vital organs can have a dramatic effect on your overall wellbeing, so it's important to keep them in good working order. Eating a healthy diet, getting some exercise, quitting smoking and keeping an eye on your alcohol intake are good places to start.

Chest Infections

Chest infections, or lower respiratory tract infections (LRTIs) as doctors sometimes refer to them, affect the airways leading to the lungs (trachea and bronchi) and the lungs themselves. They tend to be more serious than infections affecting the upper respiratory tract (URTIs), such as colds and sore throats. They are also quite common, especially among elderly people and those whose immune systems are compromised, such as cancer patients. You are more likely to contract a chest infection during the autumn and winter months.

Symptoms

Chest infections can be quite difficult to diagnose. Just because you have a chesty cough doesn't necessarily mean you have a chest infection. Your doctor will need to listen to your chest with a stethoscope to tell for sure. People who have a chest infection make telltale 'crackling' sounds as they breathe in and out. You may also have the following symptoms: coughing, mucus, chest pain and fever.

Prevention

Unlike colds and sore throats, which are usually caused by viruses, chest infections can be caused by both viruses and bacteria. To avoid harmful bugs:

 Don't smoke as this irritates your lungs and makes them more prone to infections

- Wash your hands with soap and warm water often
- Avoid crowded indoor places
- Wrap up warmly in cold weather
- Eat plenty of fruit and vegetables
- Make sure you are getting enough sleep
- Take some exercise
- Avoid stress, as this can lower your immune system
- Make sure you have your flu and pneumoccocal jabs if you are invited

Treatment

- **Take a painkiller:** Painkillers like paracetamol and aspirin can lower fever and help with aches and pains.
- **Drink plenty of fluids:** This will help to prevent dehydration.
- **Rest:** Taking it easy for a while gives your immune system a chance to do its work.
- **Try a cough mixture:** Although there is little research into how effective they are, some people find them helpful.
- **See your doctor:** Your doctor can rule out any underlying conditions, organize further tests and prescribe antibiotics if you need them. It's especially important to get medical help if your symptoms become worse, if you become disorientated or you are very short of breath.

Top Tip

Cover your mouth and nose with a scarf when the weather's cold. Research shows that this slows down the rate at which viruses reproduce in your respiratory tract.

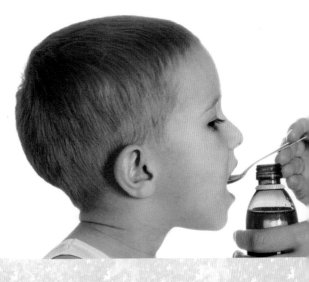

Bronchitis

Bronchitis is a lower respiratory tract infection that affects the airways leading into your lungs. It's nearly always caused by a virus – often a flu virus – which causes inflammation in the linings of your airways and makes them produce lots of mucus. Bronchitis usually clears up within a few weeks, but it can also be long lasting, especially in older people or people who already have lung problems. Symptoms include:

- ☑ **Bad cough**
- ☑ **Mucus**
- ☑ **Generally feeling unwell**
- ☑ **Aching muscles**
- ☑ **Mild fever**
- ☑ **Wheezing**
- ☑ **Shortness of breath**

Prevention and Treatment

If you fall into an at-risk category it is advisable to have an annual flu injection to prevent bronchitis. In terms of treatment, some people manage to handle their symptoms at home until they pass. Don't forget to drink plenty of fluids. However, if you are worried, do see your doctor. They may suggest:

- ☑ **A cough suppressant**: This won't clear up your symptoms, but will probably contain an antihistamine drug that causes drowsiness to give you some relief from coughing at night. You can also buy cough suppressant medicines from your local chemist.
- ☑ **An expectorant**: These are meant to help you cough up mucus, but there's no research to show that they help with bronchitis symptoms.
- ☑ **Painkillers**: These will help to bring down any fever and ease aches and pains.

Pneumonia

Pneumonia is an infection in the tiny tubes and air sacs deep inside your lungs. The infection causes them to become inflamed and fill with fluid, which makes it painful and difficult to breathe. Pneumonia is usually caused by either bacteria or viruses, and is most common in young children, elderly people and smokers. Most people make a complete recovery, but you may feel tired and lethargic for up to six weeks. Symptoms include:

- Fever
- Cough
- Mucus
- Loss of appetite

- Rapid, and sometimes irregular, heartbeat
- Shortness of breath
- Tightness in your chest
- Sharp pain in the side when you breathe

Prevention and Treatment

To prevent pneumonia, make sure you have your flu jab if you are invited, and don't smoke. There is also a vaccination against the most common form of pneumonia, pneumococcal pneumonia. This is only usually given to people with pre-existing lung or heart conditions. To treat pneumonia, cough medicines are not recommended. Instead, your doctor may suggest:

- Antibiotics to clear up any bacterial infection
- Painkillers (paracetamol, aspirin or ibuprofen) for fever and aches and pains
- Taking it easy, to help your body to recover quickly
- Plenty of fluids to help prevent dehydration caused by high fever

Chronic Obstructive Pulmonary Disease (COPD)

Chronic Obstructive Pulmonary Disease (COPD) is a disease in which the airways of the lungs have become damaged and narrowed making it difficult to breathe. Chronic bronchitis and emphysema are two conditions that lead to COPD. The main cause of all these conditions is smoking. COPD symptoms are often worse in winter and are:

- Persistent coughing, especially in the morning
- Phlegm
- Wheezing

- Shortness of breath
- Recurring chest infections (*see page 88*)
- Exhaustion

Prevention

- ☑ Don't smoke and avoid smoky environments
- ☑ Have flu vaccinations (if you are invited)
- ☑ Exercise regularly to keep your lungs healthy

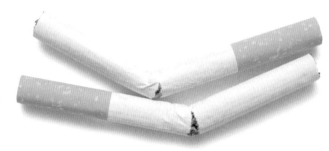

Treatment

There is no cure for COPD, but the following may help:

- ☑ **Self help**: It's important to stay as fit and active as possible, despite your breathlessness.
- ☑ **Quit smoking**: Doing so will slow down the progress of your disease.
- ☑ **Pulmonary rehabilitation**: These hospital-based programmes aim to improve your capacity for exercise, mobility and self-confidence.
- ☑ **Bronchodilators**: These inhalers relax the airways and make breathing easier.
- ☑ **Theophylline tablets**: Like bronchodilators, these make the airways relax and open up.
- ☑ **Steroids**: Your doctor may prescribe these if your symptoms become severe.
- ☑ **Antibiotics**: For any lung infections you may develop.
- ☑ **Oxygen**: Some people with COPD may benefit from having oxygen at home.

Angina

Angina is a pain or discomfort in the chest, which may also spread to your arm, neck, jaw or back. People often describe the pain as a tightness or heaviness. It's caused by narrowing of the coronary arteries, which reduces the blood supply to the heart. The pain often comes on with physical activity or emotional upset. However, with what's known as 'unstable' angina, the symptoms can come on at any time. In addition to the pain, symptoms include breathlessness, fatigue and dizziness.

Prevention

- ✅ Give up smoking
- ✅ Exercise regularly
- ✅ Don't drink to excess
- ✅ Eat a well-balanced diet and try to maintain a healthy weight
- ✅ Get your cholesterol and triglyceride (another kind of fat that works in tandem with cholesterol) levels checked, and treat with medication if your doctor says they are abnormally raised
- ✅ If you are a diabetic, make sure your blood glucose is well controlled
- ✅ Heart disease can be hereditary so, if you have a close relative with angina, you are more likely to get it too – making the above actions even more crucial

> ## Top Tip
>
> If you are suffering from erectile dysfunction (ED), get this assessed, as it is a marker for more serious disease, such as heart problems and diabetes (*see pages 160–61*).

Treatment

There are a range of medical and surgical treatments for angina including:

- ✅ **Glyceryl trinitrate**: Provides swift relief from angina pain, but can give you a headache.
- ✅ **Beta blockers**: These make the heart beat slower so that less oxygen is needed.
- ✅ **Calcium channel blockers**: These drugs relax the walls of the arteries and so increase the blood supply to the heart.
- ✅ **Percutaneous coronary intervention (PCI)**: This involves putting a sausage-shaped balloon into the coronary artery and inflating it to widen the artery.
- ✅ **Coronary artery bypass graft (CABG)**: This uses a blood vessel from the leg to bypass a blockage in one or more of the heart's arteries.

Heart Failure

The term heart failure sounds terrifying but it just means that your heart is not pumping blood around your body as efficiently as it should. The many possible reasons for this include a previous heart attack, high blood pressure and heart-valve problems. Symptoms include:

- Breathlessness
- Fatigue
- Swollen feet, ankles and abdomen
- Nausea
- Loss of appetite

Prevention

- Cut down on salt
- Eat a well-balanced diet
- Don't smoke
- Lead an active life
- Only drink alcohol in moderation
- Keep your stress levels down
- Keep your cholesterol and triglyceride levels down (*see* page 93)

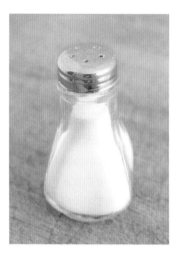

Treatment

Heart failure cannot be cured, but your symptoms can certainly be managed by adopting a healthy lifestyle and taking certain drugs, including:

- **ACE inhibitors**: These make your arteries relax, making it easier for your heart to pump blood around your body.
- **Diuretics**: Diuretics will help to reduce swelling in ankles and feet, and also breathlessness due to fluid build-up in the lungs.
- **Anticoagulants**: These will thin your blood making it less likely to clot.

Top Tip

Do not stop your doctor's medication without your doctor's advice. Sometimes even missing one day's diuretics can have ill effects. Plan ahead – if going on a coach trip, check the coach will have a toilet.

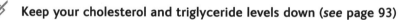

Back

Backs are something most of us take for granted – until they go wrong in some way. Having pain or immobility in your back can be extremely debilitating, especially if it prevents you from working or doing the things you enjoy. The good news is that most back conditions do get better, particularly if you try to stay positive and active.

Back pain

Back pain is distressing and disabling. So it may be annoying to hear that it's not generally considered to be a serious medical condition. There are various possible causes for back pain including sprained (pulled) muscles, slipped discs or trapped nerves. Sometimes there is no apparent cause. Most cases clear up in a few weeks.

Prevention
- Avoid lifting very heavy objects, twisting while lifting or lifting from an awkward position
- Make sure your workstation is properly assessed for health and safety
- Address stress, depression or dissatisfaction at work as these can all play a role in back pain
- Get regular exercise
- Avoid staying in one position for too long – get up, move around and stretch

Treatment
- **Stay active:** Continuing your normal daily activities is likely to give you a better outcome.
- **Take painkillers:** Try regular doses of paracetamol or ibuprofen. Doctors often advise taking both of these alternately up to the maximum permitted doses and frequencies.
- **Stretch:** Some people find gentle stretching exercises helpful.

Hot or cold packs: These may offer some relief in the short term.

 Try a therapy: Physiotherapy, osteopathy, chiropractic, massage and the Alexander technique may all help.

> # Top Tip
>
> **A hot pack is probably best for muscular pain, stiffness or discomfort, while a cold pack is better for inflammation (indicated by swelling).**

Slipped Disc

A slipped disc happens when one of the small, flexible discs between the bones of your spine starts to bulge and possibly rupture. This can put pressure on the spinal cord or nerves of the back causing serious back pain. A slipped disc normally clears up within six weeks. If it doesn't, your doctor may refer you to a back specialist. Symptoms include sharp pain in the lower back, pain on moving around and possibly pain running down one leg.

Prevention

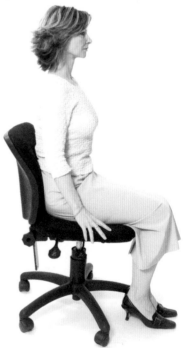

 Exercise will keep your discs in good shape and help you maintain a healthy weight

 Avoid lifting very heavy objects, twisting while lifting or lifting from an awkward position

 Avoid staying in one position for too long

 Keep an eye on your posture

Treatment

 Stay active: Start moving around as soon as possible as this will speed up your recovery.

 Physical therapies: Many people find physiotherapy, osteopathy, the Alexander technique or chiropractic helpful.

 Medication: Paracetamol or ibuprofen taken four times a day should ease the pain. If it doesn't, your doctor can prescribe the stronger painkiller, such as codeine.

☑ **Surgery:** This is only necessary in a minority of cases. The surgeon will cut away the piece of disc that is protruding. However, this does not work for everyone.

Sciatica

Sciatica is pain that radiates down your leg from the lower back and buttocks. It happens when the sciatic nerve, which starts in the lower back, gets squashed or irritated for some reason. Pregnant women sometimes get sciatica, because of changes in their posture. Another common cause is a slipped disc (*see* page 96), but there can also be no apparent reason. Sciatica usually goes away within six weeks, but can also be long lasting. Symptoms include pain stretching from your lower back down into your buttocks and legs, numbness or weakness in the affected leg and pins and needles in the feet.

Prevention

☑ **Gentle exercise will strengthen your spine and help keep it flexible**

☑ **Keep an eye on your posture**

☑ **Sleep on a medium–firm mattress**

☑ **Avoid lifting very heavy objects, twisting while lifting or lifting from an awkward position**

☑ **Maintain a healthy weight to avoid strain caused by excess weight**

☑ **Avoid being a 'completer finisher' – striving to complete a task when over tired**

Treatment

☑ **Exercise:** Try to stay physically active and return to work as soon as possible.

☑ **Painkillers:** Ibuprofen is thought to work best for sciatica. If you can't take it, try paracetamol. For severe pain, your doctor may prescribe a stronger painkiller, such as codeine, or a muscle relaxant, such as diazepam. Sometimes amitryptiline is used, as although at high doses it is used for depression, at a lower dose it can help nerve pain.

 Hot or cold packs: You may find it helpful to use one type of pack after another.

Digestive System

The digestive system allows us to break down the food we eat for use in the body. It does this by moving the food through the gut, digesting it and absorbing nutrients as it goes, and then efficiently disposing of any waste matter. The digestive tract usually manages all this with us barely noticing. However, when problems do occur it can lead to unpleasant symptoms, such as vomiting, diarrhoea and pain.

Heartburn

Heartburn is discomfort caused by stomach acid leaking up into your food tube (oesophagus). It also goes by the name of gastro-oesophageal reflux disease (GORD). It happens because the valve between your stomach and oesophagus is weakened or under pressure for some reason. Heartburn is very common, and the burning sensation in your lower chest and/or sour taste in your mouth is often accompanied by symptoms of indigestion, such as belching and bloating.

Prevention

- Sit up straight during and after eating
- Avoid tight clothing round your middle
- Don't eat heavy meals late at night
- Don't smoke
- Keep your stress levels down
- Maintain a healthy weight

Treatment

- **If you are overweight, lose weight**: This will help reduce pressure on your stomach.
- **Stop smoking**: Tobacco can make heartburn symptoms worse.
- **Avoid large meals**: Have four or five small meals a day rather than three big ones, and don't eat just before bed.
- **Avoid your triggers**: Common heartburn triggers include alcohol, coffee, chocolate, tomatoes and fatty or spicy foods.

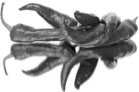

Over-the-counter remedies: These work by neutralizing stomach acid or giving the lining of the oesophagus a protective coating.

 Proton-pump inhibitors: These prescribed medicines work by reducing the amount of acid your stomach produces.

 Give the acid a little help: Raise the head of your bed to encourage stomach acid to flow downwards. Don't use extra pillows as this can increase the pressure on your stomach. Raise it up to 20 cm (8 inches) – the height recommended by gastroenterologists – gradually in order to get used to it.

Peptic Ulcer

Peptic ulcers are open sores that develop in the lining of the stomach or small intestine (duodenum). They are most common in people aged over 60 and about 25 per cent of people are thought to have one at some point. If your doctor suspects you have an ulcer they will test you for bacteria called helicobacter pylori, which is the main cause. Overuse of non-steroidal anti-inflammatory drugs (NSAIDs), such as aspirin and ibuprofen, can also be responsible. Some people have no symptoms, but signs of a peptic ulcer can include:

 Recurrent pain just below your breastbone   **Pain may wake you at night**

 Pain starts after a meal   **Blood-stained vomit**

Prevention

 Use paracetamol rather than aspirin or ibuprofen

 Cut down your tea and coffee intake

 Keep your stress levels down

 Quit smoking

 Limit alcohol.

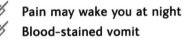

Treatment

 Antibiotics: These will kill off any helicobacter pylori in the stomach or small intestine.

- **Proton-pump inhibitors PPIs:** These reduce acid production in your stomach allowing the ulcer to heal.
- **H2 blockers:** Like PPIs these reduce the amount of acid produced by the stomach.
- **Stepping down NSAIDs:** The NSAIDs dosage is reduced at the same time as being given medication to heal the ulcer.

Did You Know?

Consuming milk and milk-based foods, such as yoghurt, is believed to 'line' the stomach and neutralize the harmful effects of stomach acid.

Diarrhoea

Diarrhoea hits us all at some point. Often it is just the natural outcome of eating too much high-fibre food or of anxiety. Sometimes, though, it's the result of an infection. People often joke about diarrhoea, but it can be extremely debilitating, not to mention dehydrating. It can also be a symptom of some quite serious conditions, such as salmonella or irritable bowel syndrome, so deserves to be taken seriously. Symptoms are:

- **Opening your bowels more than three times in one day**
- **Loose, watery stools**
- **Abdominal cramps**
- **Fever**

Prevention
- **Practise good hygiene in your kitchen to avoid food-borne infections**
- **Avoid raw or lightly cooked meat and eggs**
- **Be cautious about what you eat and drink if you travel abroad**

Treatment
- **Fluids:** Make sure you have plenty of water, juice or herbal teas to replace lost fluids.

Oral rehydration solution (ORS): This replaces lost salts and minerals and is available from all chemists.

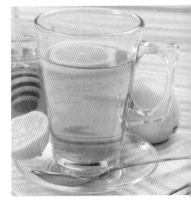

Anti-diarrhoeal drugs: Again, these are available from the chemist and can help to reduce how often you go to the toilet.

Antibiotics: If you urgently need to stop the symptoms of diarrhoea – for example, if you are on an important business trip – a course of antibiotics can help. Speak to your doctor before you go.

See your doctor: Diarrhoea that lasts for more than 10 days or blood in your stools both need medical attention.

Constipation

If you open your bowels less than three times a week you are probably constipated. The two groups of people most likely to be constipated are young women and the elderly. Sometimes medications, such as iron pills, can cause constipation. Repeatedly ignoring the urge to go to the toilet is another common cause. So are inactivity and a lack of fluids and fibre in your diet. Symptoms include:

- **Dry, hard or lumpy stools**
- **Stools that are too big or too small to pass comfortably**
- **Feeling that you can't completely empty your bowel**
- **Stomach ache**
- **Feeling bloated**

Prevention

- **Eat plenty of fibre-rich foods, such as fruit, vegetables, brown rice and wholemeal bread**
- **Drink about 10 glasses or mugs of fluid a day (but not too much tea, coffee or cola)**
- **Exercise regularly**
- **Always go to the toilet when you need to**

Treatment

If your symptoms persist despite self-help measures, your doctor may suggest:

- **Laxatives:** These should only be taken in the short term as long-term use can make the problem worse.
- **Biofeedback:** In severe cases, doctors use this technique to help people re-learn how to use their muscles to empty their bowels properly.

Appendicitis

The appendix is a small tube-like structure attached to your gut in the bottom right-hand side of your abdomen. Appendicitis is an infection of the appendix. There isn't always an obvious cause for these infections, but sometimes the appendix gets obstructed by hardened faeces. Infection sets in causing inflammation and swelling. Appendicitis should always be treated as a medical emergency. Left untreated, the appendix can burst (perforate) and cause a life-threatening infection in the lining of the abdomen (peritonitis) or blood (sepsis). Symptoms include:

- **Stomach pain that eventually settles in the lower right-hand side of your abdomen**
- **Pain is worse with pressure and on coughing or walking**
- **Loss of appetite**
- **Nausea and vomiting**
- **Mild fever**
- **Constipation or diarrhoea**

Prevention and Treatment

To prevent appendicitis eat plenty of fibre – appendicitis is less common in countries where

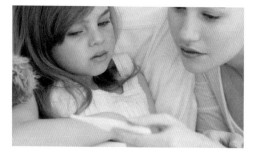

people eat a high-fibre diet. To treat it, in mild cases, doctors may be able to prescribe antibiotics. However, in most cases surgery is needed to remove the appendix. Doctors are increasingly using keyhole surgery (where instruments are passed through small incisions in your stomach wall) to do this. Living without an appendix shouldn't cause you any problems.

Did You Know?

Recent research suggests that the appendix may provide a home for 'friendly' bacteria that aid digestion and help fight infection in the gut.

Coeliac Disease

Coeliac disease affects about one in 100 people. It is an autoimmune disease (where the body's immune system attacks its own tissues). In people with coeliac disease this immune reaction is triggered by gluten, a protein found in wheat, rye and barley. Over time the body's response to gluten damages the lining of the small intestines so that it cannot absorb food properly. Coeliac disease sometimes runs in families. Symptoms vary from person to person, but can include:

- Bloating
- Pains in the stomach
- Nausea
- Diarrhoea and/or constipation
- Wind
- Heartburn and indigestion
- Weight loss
- Anaemia
- Fatigue

Prevention and Treatment

The cause of coeliac disease is unknown, although there may be a genetic factor. It cannot be prevented. There is also no cure for coeliac disease, but the symptoms can be controlled by eating a strict gluten-free diet. It's important to get a medical diagnosis before you adopt a gluten-free diet. Once you are diagnosed:

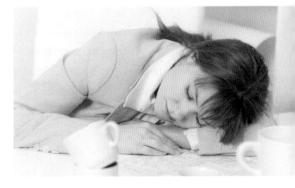

☑ **See a dietician:** Your dietician will help you to draw up a step-by-step plan to exclude gluten from your diet.

☑ **Ask about prescribed foods:** People with coeliac disease can sometimes get gluten-free foods on prescription.

☑ **Start checking labels:** Most supermarkets carry a range of gluten-free foods. Foods that contain gluten must also be clearly labelled.

☑ **Be patient:** It may take up to two years for your gut to recover.

Food poisoning

Food poisoning is an umbrella term for the various infections caused by harmful bacteria, viruses and parasites in food. You can pick up these infections by eating infected foods or by coming into contact with infected people. As anyone who's had it knows, the symptoms of food poisoning can be extremely unpleasant. In rare cases, food-borne infections can even be fatal. Symptoms include:

☑ **Nausea and vomiting**   ☑ **Diarrhoea**
☑ **Abdominal cramps**   ☑ **Fever**
                               ☑ **Dehydration**

Prevention

☑ Always wash your hands before preparing food, after touching raw food and after going to the toilet

☑ In the kitchen, keep worktops, chopping boards and utensils clean

☑ Change dishcloths and towels regularly

☑ Always cook food till it's piping hot all the way through

☑ Don't reheat food more than once

☑ Keep raw meat in sealed containers at the bottom of your fridge

☑ Make sure your fridge temperature is between 0°C and 5°C

☑ Consider whether all of the above will have been adhered to when eating food prepared outside the home...

Treatment

- ☑ **Fluids**: Plenty of drinks are always the first line of treatment for diarrhoea and vomiting. You may also want to try oral rehydration solution (ORS) which replaces lost salts and minerals (available from chemists).
- ☑ **Stop it spreading**: Wash your hands regularly to avoid passing germs on to other people.
- ☑ **See your doctor**: If diarrhoea and vomiting last for more than a few days, see your doctor.

Haemorrhoids

Haemorrhoids, or piles, are blood vessels in and around your anus that have become swollen and inflamed. They are caused by an increase in pressure in the blood vessels, perhaps because of excess weight or repeated straining when going to the loo. There is also a familial tendency to piles. About 50 per cent of people experience them at some time in their life. Symptoms include:

- ☑ **Itchiness and soreness around your back passage**
- ☑ **Bleeding and/or passing mucus after opening your bowels**
- ☑ **Pain when passing a stool**
- ☑ **Feeling as though you can't empty your bowels properly**

Prevention

- ☑ **Eat a fibre-rich diet and drink plenty of fluids to prevent constipation**
- ☑ **Exercise regularly**
- ☑ **Maintain a healthy weight**

Treatment

- ☑ **Self help**: Sitting in a bath of warm water can ease any pain, as can holding a cold pack against your back passage.
- ☑ **Laxatives**: Bulk-forming laxatives can soften your stools.
- ☑ **Creams and suppositories**: Preparations to ease your symptoms are available both over the counter and on prescription.

- **Banding**: Your doctor can place a rubber band around the base of haemorrhoids so that they decrease in size.
- **Sclerotherapy**: This involves injecting a chemical around the blood vessels in your anus to shrink your haemorrhoids.
- **Infrared coagulation**: Infrared light is used to cut off the circulation to small internal haemorrhoids.
- **Cryotherapy**: This is where the piles are frozen and so shrink back.
- **Surgery**: Surgery is often used to remove haemorrhoids that are very large.

Diverticular Disease and Diverticulitis

Sometimes small pouches, known as diverticula, can develop in the walls of your large intestine (colon). These don't cause any symptoms in most people, but some people suffer unpleasant symptoms, such as pain, constipation and diarrhoea. This is called diverticular disease. Other people get a related condition called diverticulitis, in which the diverticula become infected and inflamed. Not eating enough fibre is thought to be the cause of both conditions.

Symptoms of Diverticular Disease

- **Intermittent pain in lower abdomen, usually in the lower, left-hand side**
- **Diarrhoea or constipation**
- **Blood in stools**

Symptoms of Diverticulitis

- **Severe, constant pain in lower abdomen**
- **Fever**
- **Pain on weeing**
- **Nausea**
- **Constipation**
- **Blood in stools**

Prevention and Treatment

Getting plenty of fibre in your diet may help prevent diverticular disease and improve symptoms once you have it. For diverticular disease, a high-fibre diet can sometimes relieve your symptoms within a matter of days; over-the-counter painkillers such as paracetamol should be enough to ease any pain; avoid aspirin and ibuprofen as they may aggravate your symptoms; and bulk-forming laxatives will help if you are experiencing constipation. For diverticulitis antibiotics can be prescribed to treat the infection and painkillers such as paracetamol should help to ease the pain.

Irritable Bowel Syndrome (IBS)

Irritable bowel syndrome (IBS) is one of the most common disorders to affect the gut: somewhere between 10 and 20 per cent of people have it. It causes a wide range of symptoms, including abdominal pain, bloating and wind. The symptoms of IBS can come and go, being very acute at times and almost non-existent at others. Symptoms include:

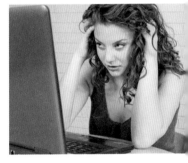

- **Abdominal pain that is relieved by opening your bowels**
- **Bloating and wind**
- **Changes in bowel habit (such as needing to get to the loo more urgently than before)**
- **Passing mucus from your back passage**
- **Symptoms are worse after eating**

Prevention and Treatment

- **Keep your stress levels down**: There is a known link between stress and IBS.
- **Self help**: It helps to eat regular meals and drink plenty of fluids. Stay active, but make time to relax, too.
- **See a dietician**: Your doctor may recommend this if he feels you may benefit from removing certain foods from your diet.
- **Anti–spasmodics**: These drugs help to reduce painful spasms in your gut.
- **Laxatives and anti-diarrhoea medication**: Your doctor will show you how to balance these so that you can go to the toilet comfortably.
- **Gut directed hypnotherapy**: This is a special kind of hypnotherapy developed for people who have IBS and other gut disorders. Ask your doctor for more information.

Urinary Tract

The urinary tract consists of your kidneys, ureters (the tubes taking urine from your kidneys to your bladder), bladder, urethra (the tube through which urine leaves your body) and, in men, the penis. The kidneys remove a waste product called urea from your blood and mix it with water to make urine. Although urine is sterile, bacteria can get into any part of the urinary tract and cause an infection.

Urinary Tract Infections (UTIs)

Urinary tract infections (UTIs) happen when bacteria get into your urinary system. They usually get in via the urethra, which is the tube that carries urine out of your body from your bladder. Infections of the lower urinary system (urethra and bladder) are much more common and are sometimes called cystitis.

UTIs are also much more common in women. About half of all women have a UTI at some point in their life. This is probably because women only have a short distance between the opening of the urethra and their bladder, making it easier for germs to enter the urinary tract. Occasionally, certain contraceptive methods, such as the cap or condoms, can cause infections. If this happens, talk to your doctor.

Symptoms

Symptoms of a lower UTI include:

- Pain, or a burning sensation, on weeing
- Needing to wee frequently or urgently
- Cloudy, bloody or smelly urine
- Pain in your lower abdomen
- Mild fever

Symptoms of an upper UTI can also include:

- High fever
- Shivering
- Nausea or vomiting
- Pain in the small of your back or side

Prevention

- Drink plenty of fluids to help flush bacteria through your urinary tract
- Wash your genitals every day and before having sex
- Always go to the toilet as soon as you get the urge
- Always wipe from front to back after going to the toilet
- Go for a wee after having sex
- Drink one or two glasses of cranberry juice a day – there's some evidence that it helps to flush bacteria through your urinary tract.

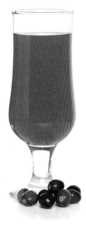

Treatment

If your symptoms have only just started it may help to drink plenty of water to try and flush any bacteria out of your system. If they persist, seek medical help.

- **Antibiotics**: A short course of antibiotics is usually effective for both lower and upper UTIs. Occasionally, the bacteria causing the infection are resistant to the antibiotic you have been given and you may need to take a course of different antibiotics.
- **Over-the-counter remedies**: These will help to relieve your symptoms, but won't clear up the infection.

Did You Know?

Constipation can increase your chances of developing a UTI. Eating more fibre and drinking plenty of fluids can help prevent it.

Urinary Incontinence

Urinary incontinence is when you wee without meaning to, and it's a much more common problem in women than men. Stress incontinence, where you leak urine on coughing, sneezing or laughing, is usually caused by weak pelvic floor muscles. Urge incontinence is when you feel the need to wee both urgently and often, and often need to get up during the night to go to the loo.

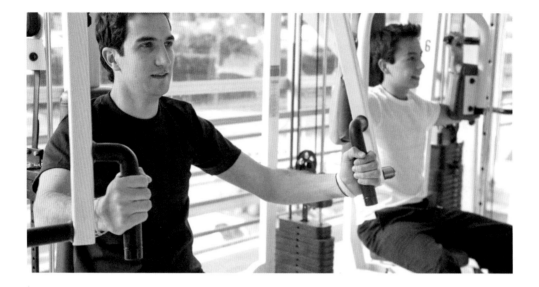

Prevention

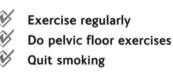

- Maintain a healthy weight
- Avoid constipation (*see* page 101)
- Cut down on alcohol and caffeine
- Exercise regularly
- Do pelvic floor exercises
- Quit smoking

Treatment for Stress Incontinence

- **Pelvic floor exercises**: These will strengthen the muscles that support your bladder.
- **Surgery**: There are several surgical procedures for stress incontinence. Your doctor will discuss your options with you.

Treatment for Urge Incontinence

- **Bladder training**: This will help you to increase the length of time between feeling the urge to wee and actually doing so.
- **Drugs**: There are medications available that reduce your urge to go to the loo.
- **Surgery**: There are a range of surgical techniques that can help.
- **Botox**: This involves injecting your bladder with botulinum toxin A to reduce your urge to wee.

Kidney Stones

Kidney stones can be extremely painful and distressing. They are solid lumps that can form in your kidneys out of substances found in urine (usually calcium). Some kidney stones stay in your body causing no problems. Others pass out in your urine. Occasionally, though, they get stuck in one of your ureters (the tubes that take urine from the kidneys to the bladder) causing intense pain.

Symptoms

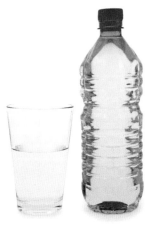

- ✔ **Sudden pain in your back or side**
- ✔ **Feeling sweaty**
- ✔ **Blood in your urine**
- ✔ **Needing to wee more often**
- ✔ **Burning sensation when you wee**

Prevention and Treatment

To prevent kidney stones, drink plenty of water and don't have too much salt. To treat:

- ✔ **Watch and wait**: Small stones may eventually pass out of your body, but this can take weeks.
- ✔ **Painkillers**: Your doctor will prescribe strong painkillers to ease the pain.
- ✔ **Alpha-blockers**: These drugs can help stones to pass down the ureters quicker.
- ✔ **Shock wave therapy**: If the stone won't budge, doctors may zap it with shock waves to break it into smaller pieces.
- ✔ **Percutaneous nephrolithotomy (PCNL)**: A minor operation in which the surgeon makes a cut in your back and uses a tube to remove a stone from your kidney.

Did You Know?

Foods such as chocolate, nuts, rhubarb and strawberries can increase the amount of calcium in your urine. If you have a calcium stone, you may be advised to avoid them.

Liver

The liver is situated just under your ribs on the right-hand side, and is estimated to have about 500 different functions ranging from fighting infection to converting food into energy. It's large, too, weighing about 1.8 kg (4 lb) in men and 1.3 kg (2.8 lb) in women. Unlike other parts of the body the liver ages well and, barring disease or damage, will function fully into old age.

Hepatitis

Hepatitis is inflammation of the liver. Drinking too much alcohol can cause this, as can a rare condition called autoimmune hepatitis, in which the body's own immune system attacks the liver. However, hepatitis is usually caused by a virus – the most common of which are:

- **Hepatitis A:** This is transmitted via food and water contaminated with faeces, usually in countries where standards of hygiene and sanitation are poor. Although unpleasant, most people make a full recovery.
- **Hepatitis B:** This is spread via blood and body fluids, for example, during unprotected sex. Mothers can also pass the virus to their babies during childbirth. Unlike hepatitis A, hepatitis B can cause long-term liver damage.
- **Hepatitis C:** This is spread through the exchange of blood, for example, when sharing needles. Like hepatitis B it can cause long-term damage to the liver.

Symptoms

Symptoms can take months to appear and some people never get any. However, you may experience:

- **Flu-like symtoms (tiredness, aches and pains, fever)**
- **Abdominal pain**
- **Nausea or vomiting**
- **Diarrhoea**
- **Loss of appetite**
- **Jaundice**

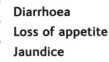

Prevention

Vaccinations against hepatitis A and hepatitis B are available. It's particularly important for people who are at risk of catching hepatitis B at work to be vaccinated. You can also protect yourself by:

- **Being cautious about where you eat when travelling in developing countries**
- **Washing your hands often, especially after going to the toilet and before preparing or eating food**
- **Always having safe sex**
- **Not sharing injecting equipment if you are an intravenous drug user**
- **Not sharing toothbrushes and razors**

Treatment

- **Hepatitis A:** There is no specific treatment for this, but you will need to avoid alcohol until you recover.
- **Hepatitis B:** Again, there is no specific treatment, but your doctor will probably advise rest, a healthy diet and no alcohol until you recover. If you develop chronic hepatitis B, you may be offered an antiviral medication called interferon.
- **Hepatitis C:** Hepatitis C is usually treated with a combination of two drugs, interferon and ribavirin.

Did You Know?

Hepatitis B is 100 times more infectious than HIV. However, there is a simple test to find out whether you have the virus and an effective vaccine to protect you against it.

Gallstones

The gall bladder is a small pouch tucked just under the liver. It stores bile, a greenish substance that helps the body to digest fat. Gallstones are solid lumps that form here. They usually look like small stones and are often made up largely of cholesterol. They are more common in overweight people (especially overweight women over 40), women who have had babies and people who have recently lost weight. Many people have no symptoms, but others may experience:

Pain just below the right ribs   Fever with shivering Vomiting
Jaundice (yellowish tinge to the skin and whites of the eyes)

Prevention and Treament

Since being overweight can be a factor, losing weight is a good preventative measure. To treat:

Watch and wait: Gallstones are often discovered by accident, perhaps during an X-ray or ultrasound scan. If your gallstones aren't actually causing you any problems, your doctor may just suggest regular scans to keep an eye on them.

Surgery: If your gallstones are causing pain and other problems, doctors may suggest removing your gall bladder using keyhole surgery. Your health won't suffer without it.

Cirrhosis

Cirrhosis is long-term scarring of the liver. Eventually the build-up of scar tissue can interfere with the blood flow through your liver and stop it functioning properly. There are various causes of cirrhosis, including drinking too much alcohol, obesity, liver infections, such as hepatitis B and C, and inherited liver conditions. Symptoms include:

Tiredness and weakness
Loss of appetite
Nausea
Build-up of fluid in the legs and abdomen

Weight loss
Tendency to bruise and bleed easily
Jaundice
Itchiness, due to a build-up of toxins
Personality changes

Prevention

Only drink alcohol in moderation
Always have safe sex to avoid liver infections
Never share injecting equipment if you are an intravenous drug user
If you are at risk of catching hepatitis B at work, get vaccinated

Treatment

Cirrhosis cannot be cured, but treatment can slow its progress by:

 Getting rid of infections: The most important are hepatitis B and hepatitis C.

Stopping bleeding: Because blood cannot pass through the liver efficiently, veins above the liver may become dilated and even burst. Drugs, such as beta blockers, can help reduce pressure in these veins. They can also be sealed with rubber bands to stop bleeding.

Reducing fluid: A low-salt diet combined with diuretic drugs will help to reduce fluid in the abdomen and ankles.

Checklist

 Don't smoke: Or, if you do smoke, quit – to prevent damage to your lungs and lower your risk of chest infections.

Try to eat a healthy well-balanced diet: Keeping salt and cholesterol to a minimum will help to keep your heart healthy, while plenty of fibre will ward off digestive ailments, such as constipation and diverticular disease.

Fluids: Drink plenty of non-caffeinated, non-alcoholic fluids to keep your urinary tract healthy.

Keep in shape: Exercise regularly to maintain a healthy weight and keep your heart and lungs in good shape.

Avoid too much alcohol: Drink within safe limits to protect your heart and liver.

Vaccinations: If you fall into an at-risk group for flu – if you are elderly or asthmatic, for example – make sure you take up your doctor's annual invitations for flu jabs.

Hygiene: Wash your hands regularly to lower your risk of infections, such as gastroenteritis.

Look after your back: To prevent back problems, such as slipped discs and sciatica, take care of your back.

Keep an eye on your stress levels: Stress is a factor in many health conditions including irritable bowel syndrome and back pain.

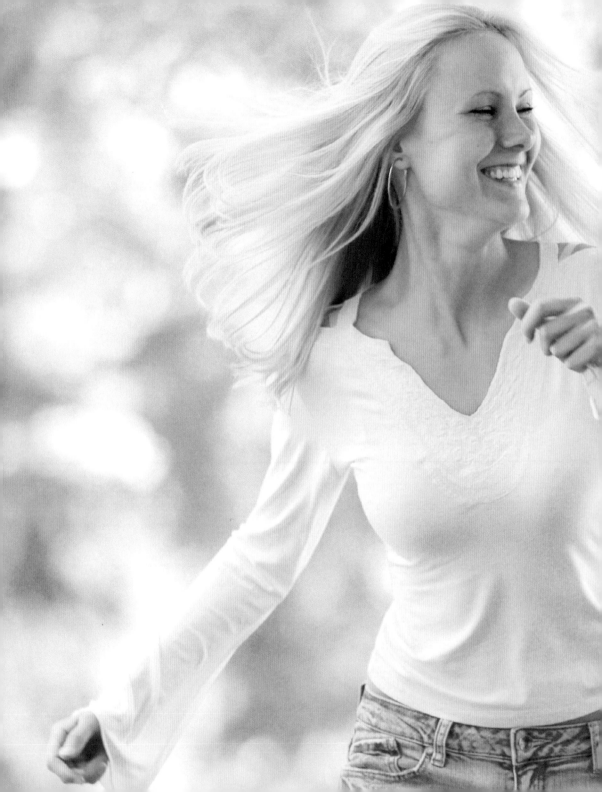

Whole Body Health

Skin

Your skin is the largest organ in your body. It has several important functions. One of these is temperature control – blood vessels under the skin dilate and contract depending on how hot you are. Your skin also forms a protective barrier against infection and stops you losing too much water. Skin is also the organ of touch, allowing us to be sensitive and responsive to our environment. Your skin is amazing – look after it.

Contact dermatitis

Contact dermatitis is skin inflammation that happens whenever your body comes into contact with a particular substance. About 75 per cent of cases of contact dermatitis affect the hands and many cases are work-associated. It's more common in women than men. There are two types of contact dermatitis: allergic and irritant.

 Allergic contact dermatitis: This happens when your skin has an allergic reaction to a substance that is normally harmless, such as nickel or latex. When you are exposed to the allergen for the first time, you become sensitized to it. After that, it causes a reaction whenever you come into contact with it. Like other allergy-related conditions, allergic contact dermatitis sometimes runs in families. Symptoms include red, inflamed, dry and blistered skin, and intense itching.

 Irritant contact dermatitis: This is more common and happens when your skin is damaged by irritants, such as detergents, perfumes or solvents. It can happen after repeated exposure to a weak irritant or after a single exposure to a strong irritant. Symptoms include red, inflamed, dry and blistered skin, and burning, stinging and soreness.

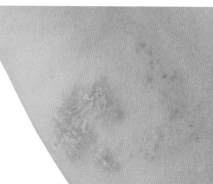

Prevention

It's difficult to predict which substances may
cause contact dermatitis, but you can take
some sensible precautions:

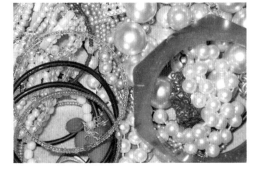

- **Avoid cheap jewellery that may
  contain nickel**
- **Wear gloves and protective
  clothing when working with
  potential irritants like detergents, solvents and adhesives**
- **Choose fragrance-free cosmetics and toiletries**

Treatment

- **Avoidance:** The first-line treatment in any case of contact dermatitis is to try and
  avoid the substance that's causing it. Your doctor or a dermatologist can help you
  identify the culprit. If it can't be avoided, wearing gloves or protective clothing may
  solve the problem.
- **Emollients:** Used regularly, moisturizing creams can help to relieve dry or cracked skin.
  Keep trying different ones until you find one that suits you. Also, you may need a
  different one for your face, say, to your legs. Some contain urea, which, although very
  good for certain skin conditions, may sting like mad on cracked skin.
- **Corticosteroids:** If necessary, your doctor can also prescribe a steroid cream to
  dampen down inflammation.

Rosacea

Rosacea usually begins with redness on the cheeks, nose, chin or forehead. Left untreated, it
can slowly worsen to include other symptoms (*see below*). It's more common in women than
men, but tends to be more serious in men. It's not known what causes rosacea, but certain
things can trigger it, including sunlight, alcohol and stress.

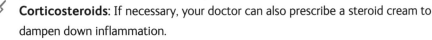

Symptoms

Symptoms of rosacea may come and go and include:

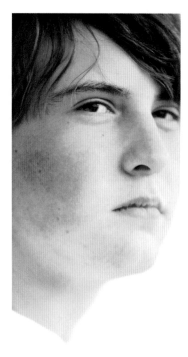

- ✔ Redness on cheeks, chin, nose and forehead
- ✔ Flushing
- ✔ Thread veins
- ✔ Acne
- ✔ Skin thickening, particularly on the nose
- ✔ Irritated or bloodshot eyes

Prevention

- ✔ Always wear sunscreen on your face (or a hat) on sunny days
- ✔ Keep your stress levels down
- ✔ Only drink alcohol in moderation
- ✔ Have warm baths rather than hot ones
- ✔ Cover your face in cold or windy weather
- ✔ Don't over-exert yourself when exercising

Treatment

You may need to have treatment for several months before you notice an improvement.

- ✔ **Creams and gels**: Metronidazole cream or gel is usually used to treat mild to moderate acne.
- ✔ **Antibiotic tablets**: Oral antibiotics, such as tetracyclines and erythromycin, may be recommended for more serious cases.
- ✔ **Laser treatment**: This can be effective for pronounced thread veins.

Did You Know?

Women of childbearing age should use a barrier method of contraception, such as condoms, while taking tetracyclines as they can cause defects in unborn babies.

Psoriasis

Psoriasis is a common condition in which skin cells reproduce too quickly. This means that dead skin cells accumulate on the skin causing scaly red patches. Psoriasis can affect anyone at any age and tends to come and go. It isn't contagious and can't be transferred from one part of the body to another. About 30 per cent of people with psoriasis have a family history of it. Elbows, knees, lower back and scalp are most commonly affected, but it can also affect the genital area in some cases, which can be particularly uncomfortable.

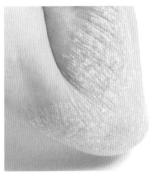

Symptoms

 Raised red patches of skin, covered with silvery-white scales

 Itching and burning

Prevention and Treatment

To prevent psoriasis avoid alcohol, cigarettes and stress, as these can all be triggers. Psoriasis cannot be cured, but can be controlled.

 Emollients: However mild or severe your psoriasis is, it's very important to moisturize your skin to keep it supple and healthy.

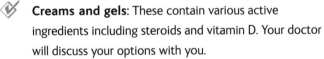 **Creams and gels**: These contain various active ingredients including steroids and vitamin D. Your doctor will discuss your options with you.

Phototherapy: Some people find exposure to ultraviolet light two or three times a week helpful.

Oral medications: There are various drugs used to treat psoriasis including methotrexate, which slows the rate at which skin cells divide, and ciclosporin, which suppresses the immune system.

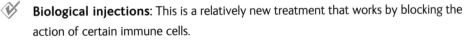 **Biological injections**: This is a relatively new treatment that works by blocking the action of certain immune cells.

Hives

Also known as nettle rash or urticaria, hives is a raised red itchy rash that can appear anywhere on the skin. It's caused by a number of different things including allergies, irritants, infections and autoimmune diseases like lupus. However, in about half of all cases no cause is found. The rash usually goes in a few days, but can also be chronic – in some cases even lasting several years.

Symptoms

 Extremely itchy rash consisting of pale, raised bumps surrounded by red skin

Rash may move around the body

Sleeplessness due to itching

Prevention and Treatment

Avoid possible triggers. These include stress, alcohol, aspirin, hot baths, strawberries, tomatoes and processed foods. To deal with hives:

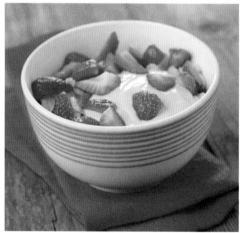

Be vigilant: Hives can sometimes be a sign of a life-threatening allergic reaction called anaphylaxis. If you have other symptoms, such as breathing difficulties or a racing heart, call 999 for an ambulance.

Antihistamines: These itch-reducing drugs are available over the counter. Try them at home and, if your symptoms don't improve in a couple of days, see your doctor.

Steroid tablets: Your doctor may prescribe a short course of these if your symptoms are severe.

Top Tip

People who have chronic hives sometimes find relaxation techniques, such as meditation or self-hypnosis, helpful for lowering their stress levels and easing their symptoms.

Hands and Feet

The hands and feet share a similar bone structure and both are controlled by a complex network of muscles and tendons. Both suffer a lot of abuse in our daily lives, and feet, in particular, can start to develop problems as we get older. The feet sometimes suffer ill effects from being squashed into shoes all day long – fungal infections, for example. Our busy hands, meanwhile, are more prone to wear and tear of the nerves and tendons.

Athlete's Foot

Athlete's foot doesn't just affect athletic types, but it is more common in boys and men. Athlete's foot is caused by fungi that normally live harmlessly on our skin. These fungi thrive in warm, dark, moist conditions, and that's why they tend to infect the skin between the toes. It's also why athlete's foot is more common in people who spend lots of time in swimming pools, showers and changing rooms. Left untreated athlete's foot can spread to the rest of the foot, including the toenails, and even other parts of the body.

Symptoms
- Itchy, red peeling skin on the feet, particularly between the toes
- Burning and stinging sensation

Prevention
- Wash your feet in cold water every day and carefully dab them dry, especially between the toes
- Alternate shoes rather than wearing the same pair every day
- Avoid wearing tight shoes
- Choose shoes made out of natural materials, such as leather or canvas

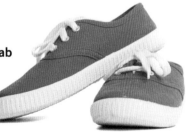

Wear cotton socks and change them daily

Wear flip-flops in showers and changing rooms

Don't wear anyone else's shoes

Treatment

It's wise to seek treatment early on, because athlete's foot is more tricky to deal with if it spreads.

Surgical spirit: This is available from your local chemist and may be enough to clear up mild cases. Dab onto affected areas with a cotton wool ball. Remember to wash your hands thoroughly afterwards.

Antifungal powder: This shouldn't be used directly on affected skin as it can be an irritant. Do dust the inside of shoes and trainers with it, though.

Antifungal creams and lotions: These are available from your pharmacist or from your doctor. The infection can persist after symptoms clear up, so follow instructions carefully. Remember to wash your hands after using them.

Antifungal tablets: Your doctor may need to prescribe these if your athlete's foot refuses to clear up.

Top Tip

Surprisingly, athlete's foot is also common in sandal wearers. This is because the skin can dry out and crack making it more vulnerable to fungal infections. If you're a regular sandal wearer, make sure you moisturize your feet often.

Verrucas

A verruca is simply a wart that grows on the sole of your foot. They are harmless, but can cause a sharp, unpleasant pain if you get one on your heel or the ball of your foot. The human papilloma virus, which causes warts and verrucas, is very contagious. It thrives in warm, moist conditions, and is often picked up in swimming pools and changing rooms.

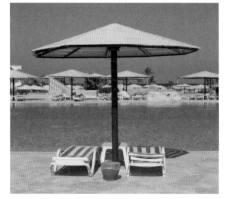

Symptoms
- Small, dark mark, which later turns grey or brown
- Rough, cauliflower-like appearance
- May develop a black spot in the middle, caused by bleeding

Prevention
- Keep your feet clean and dry
- Cover up any cuts or scratches
- Wear flip-flops in communal showers and changing rooms
- Don't share towels
- If you have a verruca, wear a verruca sock when you go swimming

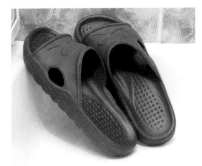

Treatment
- **Self help**: Don't be tempted to pick at your verruca. Cover it with a plaster, instead. Over-the-counter creams and gels are available. Follow the instructions carefully and see your doctor if your verruca persists or is painful.
- **Salicylic acid**: Your doctor may prescribe a preparation containing salicylic acid to kill the virus. This works well in about 75 per cent of cases.
- **Cryotherapy**: This involves freezing the verruca with liquid nitrogen or nitrous oxide.
- **Surgery**: The verruca is burned with an electric needle before being scooped out.

Ingrowing Toenails

An ingrowing toenail is one that grows sideways into the skin of the toe, causing pain and inflammation. They can be very painful indeed, especially if the skin becomes infected. Ingrowing toenails usually affect the big toe. They often happen when you cut your toenails too low at the sides. Or you may be prone to them because of the way you walk or stand. Too-tight shoes, tights and socks don't help, either.

Symptoms
- Red, swollen and tender skin next to the toenail
- Bleeding or pus if the skin becomes infected

Prevention
- Cut toenails in a straight (rather than round) line, and don't cut them too short
- Always wear well-fitting shoes, tights and socks

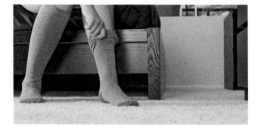

Treatment
- **Self help:** If your nail has only just started to grow into your skin, try gently massaging the skin away from the nail each day. Soak your foot in warm water first and use a little oil or foot lotion. If it gets worse, see your doctor.
- **Painkillers:** Paracetamol should help to ease the pain.
- **Surgery:** A quick, minor operation to remove the portion of nail that's digging into your toe is usually all that's needed.

Carpal Tunnel Syndrome

The carpal tunnel is a short tunnel that runs under a ridge of bones and ligament in your wrist. The median nerve, which gives sensation

Did You Know?

There's no evidence that the traditional remedy of cutting a 'V' into your nail to relieve an ingrowing toenail actually works. Always seek professional help.

and movement to your hand, runs through it. In carpal tunnel syndrome, the tunnel narrows for some reason putting pressure on the nerve. Often the cause isn't found, but you are more prone to carpal tunnel syndrome if you are pregnant, if you have a family history of it or if you have certain other conditions, such as rheumatoid arthritis and diabetes.

Symptoms

- ✔ Pain, numbness or tingling in the thumb, index finger, middle finger and half of the ring finger (if the little finger and half of the ring finger are affected, it may be compression of the ulnar nerve in the Guyon canal instead)
- ✔ Weakness and clumsiness in thumbs and fingers
- ✔ Symptoms are often worse at night

Prevention

- ✔ If your work involves doing repetitive movements with your hands (as in typing) make sure you take regular breaks
- ✔ If you are overweight, it may help to lose weight

Treatment

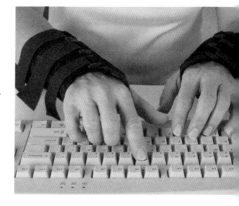

- ✔ **Self help:** Cold packs may help to relieve your symptoms, and some people find yoga beneficial.
- ✔ **Splinting:** Some people find it helpful to wear a wrist splint at night to relieve pressure on the median nerve.
- ✔ **Corticosteroids:** If splinting doesn't help, your doctor may suggest a course of steroid tablets or an injection.
- ✔ **Surgery:** In severe cases you may need surgery to widen your carpal tunnel.

Raynaud's Phenomenon

Raynaud's phenomenon is a common condition in which the small arteries in the hands are oversensitive to changes in temperature. In cold temperatures the arteries constrict and cut off the blood supply to the fingers. The feet, nose and ears are sometimes affected, too. Usually there's no known cause for Raynaud's, but it can occur in people who have other diseases, such as scleroderma, a disease affecting the connective tissue. It's also more common in women than men.

Symptoms

- ✓ Extremities turn white and then blue in cold conditions
- ✓ Extremities may go hot and red as blood returns
- ✓ Pain, numbness and tingling

Prevention

- ✓ Keep your whole body warm when the weather is cold
- ✓ Always wear gloves and warm footwear
- ✓ Consider using self-heating handwarmers (available online)
- ✓ Leave clothes you plan to wear the next day in the airing cupboard so they are warm when you put them on
- ✓ Exercise regularly
- ✓ Avoid stress if this is a trigger
- ✓ If you smoke, stop

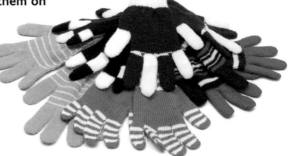

Treatment

- ✓ **Self help:** You may find that self-help measures (*see above*) are enough to manage your symptoms.
- ✓ **Vasodilators:** These are drugs that open up the small blood vessels. You will need to work with your doctor to find the one that suits you best.

Did You Know?

Viagra-like drugs taken on a regular basis have been shown to be beneficial against Raynaud's, but seek help from your doctor before trying anything. Also, the drug companies do not yet have a licence for treating this condition.

Blood and Circulation

Blood is constantly circulating throughout your body. It carries nutrients and oxygen to your body's tissues and also removes waste products. Your blood is pumped around your circulatory system by your heart. The blood vessels that carry oxygen-rich blood (which is bright red) to the tissues are called arteries, while the vessels that return deoxygenated blood (blueish) to the lungs are called veins. Problems can occur with the blood itself and also the complex system that carries it around the body.

High Blood Pressure (Hypertension)

High blood pressure happens when the walls of your arteries lose their flexibility or become narrowed, perhaps because of eating too much salt or drinking too much alcohol. This means the blood can't flow freely through them. Hypertension isn't an illness as such, but it needs addressing as it can lead to serious health problems, such as heart attacks, strokes and kidney failure. The higher your blood pressure, the shorter your life expectancy. Taking steps to reduce your blood pressure will reduce your risk of heart attacks and other serious health problems. It may also have spin-off benefits, such as losing weight and feeling more energetic.

Symptoms

You probably won't have any symptoms if your blood pressure is high. The only way to tell is to have your blood pressure measured by a nurse or doctor. Although symptoms are rare, a few people may have:

- Headaches
- Breathlessness
- Nosebleeds
- Erectile dysfunction (ED)

Prevention

To keep your blood pressure down:

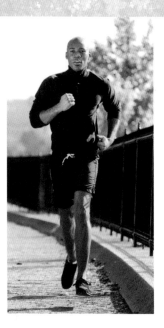

- **Quit smoking** – tobacco is one of the biggest risk factors for high blood pressure
- **Stay active** – moderate activity, such as brisk walking or cycling; 30 minutes a day is plenty
- **Try to maintain a healthy weight.**
- **Cut down your salt intake**
- **Eat more fruit and vegetables**
- **Only drink alcohol in moderation**
- **Keep your cholesterol and triglyceride levels down**

Treatment

If your blood pressure stays high despite lifestyle changes, your doctor will probably suggest medication to bring it down. What kind you have depends on your age, race and how high your blood pressure is.

- **ACE inhibitors**: These work by relaxing the walls of the arteries. You will probably be offered them if you are under 55 and are not African-Caribbean.
- **Calcium channel blockers**: Like ACE inhibitors, these relax the walls of the arteries. They are normally prescribed if you are over 55 or if you are African-Caribbean.
- **Beta-blockers**: These are sometimes used with other blood pressure medications to bring the blood pressure down further.
- **Diuretics**: These help the body get rid of salts and fluids.

Top Tip

Not only are fruit and veg packed with fibre and vitamins, they are also a good source of potassium, which balances out the negative effects of salt.

Varicose Veins

Varicose veins are very common: nearly one third of women get these swollen veins in their legs or feet at some point, and about 15 per cent of men. They are caused by weak or damaged valves in your veins. Normally these one-way valves stop blood running back down your legs, but weakened valves allow blood to seep backwards and pool in the veins. Eventually the veins become enlarged and lumpy or 'varicose'. Symptoms include:

- **Swollen dark-purple or blue veins, usually in the legs or feet**
- **Aching, heavy legs**
- **Swollen feet and ankles**

Prevention
- **Don't stand for long periods**
- **Exercise regularly to keep your blood moving**
- **Maintain a healthy weight**

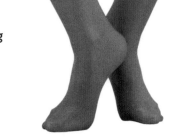

Treatment
- **Self help:** Wear compression tights or stockings to stop your varicose veins getting any worse.
- **Surgery:** There are several different surgical techniques used to treat varicose veins. The most common is ligation and stripping. This involves tying off the top of affected veins then stripping them out through an incision lower down your leg. (Note: many areas of the UK do not fund surgery for varicose veins.)
- **Endovenous laser therapy:** A laser is used to cauterize the affected veins and seal them off.
- **Sclerotherapy:** This involves injecting your veins with a chemical that damages them and causes them to close up.

Top Tip

Put compression tights or stockings on before you get out of bed in the morning and before your veins have a chance to bulge.

Anaemia

Anaemia is a lack of a red oxygen-carrying substance called haemoglobin in the blood. This can happen for various reasons, but the most common is a lack of iron. Iron is a vital component of haemoglobin and, without it, iron-deficiency anaemia can develop. A poor diet, heavy periods or internal bleeding – from a stomach ulcer, for example – can all make you deficient in iron. Pregnancy can cause iron deficiency, too, because of extra demands for iron from your baby. Symptoms include:

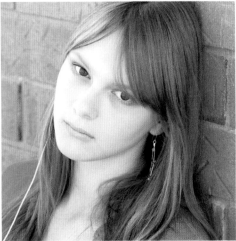

- Tiredness and lethargy
- Pale skin
- Abnormally smooth tongue
- Shortness of breath
- Heart palpitations

Prevention

- **Make sure you eat lots of iron-rich foods, including lean red meat, green leafy vegetables, beans, lentils, prunes and fortified breakfast cereals**
- **If your periods are very heavy, see your doctor**

Treatment

Before treating you, your doctor will try to work out the underlying cause of your anemia. Your doctor will usually give you iron tablets to bring your iron levels up. These can have side effects, such as heartburn and constipation. It may help to take them just after meals.

Top Tip

Drinking a vitamin C-rich drink like orange juice with meals helps your body to absorb iron from foods. This is especially useful for vegetarians because our bodies can't absorb the iron in plants (the 'ferric' form of iron) as easily as that in meat (the 'ferrous' form).

Stroke

Strokes occur when the blood supply to the brain is interrupted. They can destroy or damage brain cells that control important functions in the body, such as movement and speech. Anyone can have a stroke, but you are more likely to have one if you smoke or have high blood pressure. It can take many months to recover from a stroke. A stroke is an emergency. *If you think you or someone else may be having a stroke, call the emergency services (999, or 911 if you are in the US for example) for an ambulance.* See page 236 for more information on symptoms and dealing with a stroke in an emergency.

Prevention

- Stop smoking
- Have your blood pressure checked regularly
- Take regular exercise
- Cut down on salty and fatty foods
- Get your cholesterol and triglyceride levels measured, treating if necessary
- Eat lots of fruit and vegetables
- Keep an eye on your alcohol intake

Treatment

Treatment for ischaemic strokes may include:

- **Anticoagulants (thrombolytics):** These 'clot-busting' drugs help to break down any clots.
- **Blood pressure medication:** You may be given diuretics and ACE inhibitors (*see* High blood pressure, page 129) to bring your blood pressure down.
- **Statins:** To remove cholesterol from your blood.
- **Surgery:** To remove any blockages or blood in the brain, or to repair any burst blood vessels.

Leukaemia

Leukaemia is a cancer of the white blood cells. In people with leukaemia, the white blood cells become abnormal. Because the body doesn't have enough normal white blood cells, the immune system doesn't work properly. People who have it may also become anaemic and have problems with blood clotting. Leukaemia is often thought of as a childhood cancer, but in fact it affects three times as many adults as children. There are two main types of leukaemia: acute – in which symptoms come on rapidly and aggressively – and chronic, where symptoms develop slowly. Symptoms include:

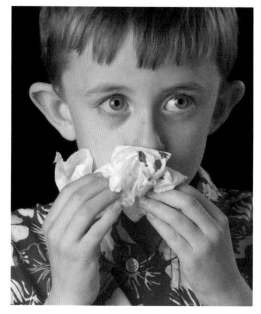

- Pale skin
- Fatigue
- Breathlessness
- Repeated infections
- Bleeding gums or nosebleeds
- Easily bruised skin
- Swollen glands

Prevention and Treatment

The main piece of preventative advice is to not smoke – smoking is a known risk factor for many cancers. If you are diagnosed with leukaemia, you will be cared for by what's known as a multi-disciplinary team, or MDT. This is a group of health professionals who have different skills. They'll help you come up with a treatment plan that may include:

- **Blood transfusions**: To give your body more healthy white blood cells.
- **Chemotherapy**: To kill the abnormal cells.
- **Stem cell transplant**: If you don't respond to chemotherapy, an infusion of stem cells may 'kickstart' your body into producing normal white blood cells.

Bones, Muscles and Joints

Our bones, muscles and joints are what keep us active and mobile. They are involved in every single movement that we make. Our bones alone are a miracle of engineering. They're very light, but at the same time strong enough to support our weight. Joints are where two bones meet. They give our bodies flexibility. Muscles, meanwhile, pull on the joints to make them work. When we develop problems with our bones, muscles or joints it often leads to a loss of mobility and flexibility.

Arthritis

Arthritis simply means inflammation of the joints. There are two main types of arthritis: osteoarthritis and rheumatoid arthritis. Osteoarthritis is the most common kind – damage to the protective cartilage in the joints leads to inflammation and changes in the bone structure. Osteoarthritis most often affects the knees, hips or hands. Rheumatoid arthritis is another, less common, form of arthritis in which the body's immune system attacks the joints so that they become damaged and inflamed. Rheumatoid arthritis often starts in the hands and feet, but may spread to other parts of the body.

Symptoms

The symptoms for osteoarthritis are:

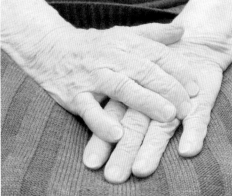

 Pain
 Stiffness, especially in the morning
 Loss of strength in the affected part
 Enlarged 'knobbly' joints

With rheumatoid arthritis you
may also experience:

 Swelling and redness around
affected joints
 Joints may be warm to the touch
 Loss of appetite
 Generally feeling tired and unwell

Top Tip

Lots of people with arthritis find capsaicin, which is derived from chillis, helpful for relieving pain. Creams and gels containing capsaicin are widely available. Just rub them onto the painful area three or four times a day. But wash your hands afterwards, as it can be very painful if you get it near your eyes or genitals!

Prevention

 Try to maintain a healthy weight
 Exercise regularly to strengthen your muscles
 Take care of your joints – avoid too much weight-bearing activity, such as running and weight training

Treatment

 Paracetamol: This may be all you need to control any pain.
 Non-steroidal anti-inflammatory drugs (NSAIDs): If paracetamol doesn't help, your doctor may prescribe a painkiller that reduces inflammation as well as relieving pain, such as ibuprofen.
 Steroid injections: These are very effective at reducing pain and inflammation, but can only be used in the short term.
 Physiotherapy: Physiotherapy can help you to manage everyday tasks and stay mobile.
 Surgery: This may be minor – to repair damaged cartilage, for example – or a full joint replacement.

For rheumatoid arthritis your doctor may also suggest:

 Disease modifying anti-rheumatic drugs (DMARDs): These dampen down the immune system's attack on the joints.

Biologic drugs: These are a new kind of drug that offer good control of rheumatic arthritis symptoms for some people.

Gout

Gout is a disorder that causes painful attacks of inflammation in the joints. It usually affects the big toe joint. The attacks are sparked by high levels of uric acid in the blood. Contrary to popular belief, gout isn't necessarily caused by high living. It can be linked to a high-protein diet and too much alcohol, but can actually affect anyone of any age. It's most common in people who are overweight, men over the age of 30 and people who have a family history of it.

Symptoms

- Excruciating pain in the joint
- Skin may be red and shiny
- Mild fever
- Loss of appetite
- Tiredness

Prevention

- Avoid red meat, game and seafood, as these can raise uric acid levels in the body
- Cut down your intake of beer, port, red wine and sugary soft drinks as these can also raise uric acid levels
- If you are overweight, lose weight

Treatment

- **Non-steroidal anti-inflammatory drugs (NSAIDs)**: These are usually the first-line treatment for gout as they help to reduce inflammation as well as relieving pain.
- **Allopurinol**: If the amount of uric acid in your blood stays high despite lifestyle changes, you may need to take this drug on a long-term basis to reduce your uric acid levels.

Did You Know?

Crash or 'yo-yo' dieting increases your risk of gout as it encourages the kidneys to retain more uric acid.

Osteoporosis

Our bones are made of a solid outer layer and a porous inner layer that resembles dense honeycomb. As we get older our bones naturally lose density. In osteoporosis they get so porous that they become fragile and prone to fractures. Lots of factors can cause this, but in particular not eating enough calcium or doing enough vigorous exercise early in life. Often the first sign of osteoporosis is a fracture: one in two women and one in five men over the age of 50 will break a bone at some point.

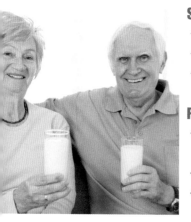

Symptoms
- ✔ Fractures, especially of the wrist, hip or spine
- ✔ Joint pains
- ✔ Difficulty standing or sitting up straight

Prevention
- ✔ Do plenty of weight-bearing exercise like weight training or aerobics in your teens and twenties
- ✔ Continue doing gentle exercise into old age
- ✔ Eat plenty of calcium-rich foods, such as milk, green leafy vegetables and tinned sardines
- ✔ Expose your skin to gentle sunlight to build up your vitamin D levels.
- ✔ Don't smoke and don't drink too much alcohol
- ✔ If you are a man, get your testosterone level checked as low levels can increase the risk of osteoporosis

Treatment
- ✔ **High-dose calcium and vitamin D supplements:** Taking these helps to reduce the risk of fractures.
- ✔ **Bisphosphonates:** These drugs are often prescribed for post-menopausal women to slow down the rate of bone loss.

Did You Know?
A man's testosterone level is at its highest at about 9 a.m.

Hormone replacement therapy (HRT): This can help menopausal symptoms as well as maintaining bone density.

Frozen Shoulder

A frozen shoulder happens when the tissues around your shoulder joint tighten so much that you can't move it freely. The medical name for frozen shoulder (if you want to impress your friends!) is adhesive encapsulitis. Usually there's no obvious explanation, but it may follow a shoulder injury or heart attack. Frozen shoulder is also more common in people who are diabetic. It can take several years to recover completely.

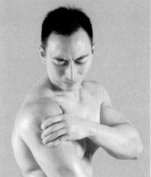

Symptoms
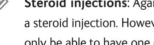 **Pain in the shoulder, particularly at night**
Very restricted movement

Prevention and Treatment
Sadly, there is no way to prevent frozen shoulder, but treatment can include:

Painkillers: If your symptoms are quite mild, a simple painkiller, such as paracetamol, may be all you need. If your pain is severe, your doctor may suggest an anti-inflammatory painkiller, such as ibuprofen. This will help to reduce inflammation in your shoulder too.

Steroid injections: Again, if your symptoms are severe, your doctor may recommend a steroid injection. However, too many can damage your shoulder more, so you may only be able to have one or two.

Physiotherapy: Your physiotherapist can help you explore a number of options to help increase your shoulder mobility and ease pain, including hot or cold packs, transcutaneous electrical nerve stimulation (TENS) and massage.

Surgery: If other treatments fail, you may be referred for keyhole surgery to remove scar tissue and release your shoulder joint.

Tennis Elbow

Tennis elbow doesn't just affect tennis players. In fact it's more likely to strike people who make repetitive movements with their arms during the course of their work, such as plasterers and carpenters. It happens when the tendons attached to the knobbly bit on the outside of your elbow become inflamed. It's not difficult to diagnose and can usually be treated by your family doctor.

Symptoms

- Pain or tenderness on the outside of your elbow
- Pain is made worse by gripping or twisting movements
- Possibly pain in your forearm

Prevention and Treatment

If you are prone to or at risk of tennis elbow, certain stretching or warming up techniques may help, along with strapping of the forearm, but there is little evidence to show how useful these measures are. Tennis elbow should resolve itself given time and rest. If possible, cut out all repetitive movements with the affected arm for a while. If it doesn't resolve itself, your doctor may suggest:

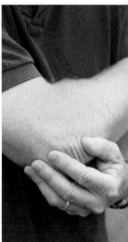

- **Painkillers**: Paracetamol should be all you need.
- **Anti-inflammatory gel**: This is available from your chemist, and some people find it helpful to rub it onto the affected area 3–4 times a day. You can increase the levels of gel getting into the skin by covering it with clingfilm for a couple of hours (but no longer to avoid soggy skin).
- **Steroid injection**: These are very effective for relieving pain, but overuse can do more harm than good.
- **Physiotherapy**: If the pain carries on for a long time, physiotherapy may help to ease it.

Did You Know?

A similar condition – golfer's elbow – can affect the bony projection on the inside of your elbow. As with tennis elbow, it's not restricted to golfers.

Metabolism

Metabolism is the word used to describe all the biochemical processes that go on inside our bodies. At any one time there are thousands of metabolic processes working away in our bodies. Breaking down the food we eat into energy is just one. We usually remain fairly oblivious to all this activity – until, that is, something goes wrong.

Diabetes

In diabetes the glucose levels in the blood are too high. This is due to a lack of insulin, the hormone that normally breaks glucose down into energy. Either the body doesn't produce enough insulin or the insulin is does produce doesn't work properly. Left untreated, diabetes will eventually lead to unconsciousness and even death. In the long term, poorly controlled diabetes can cause serious complications, including heart attacks, strokes and blindness. There are two types of diabetes: type 1 and type 2.

 Type 1: This occurs when the body's insulin-making cells have been completely destroyed, so that the body can't produce any insulin at all. Nobody knows why this happens. Type 1 usually appears in childhood or the teenage years.

Type 2: This type of diabetes is more common and usually develops later in life. The body stops producing enough insulin or the insulin it produces doesn't work properly. People who are overweight or who have high blood pressure are more at risk of developing type 2 diabetes.

Symptoms

Type 1 symptoms tend to come on rapidly. In Type 2 they usually develop gradually. They are:

Did You Know?

There are now some children developing type 2 diabetes due to dietary factors and obesity.

- ✓ Extreme thirst
- ✓ Fatigue
- ✓ Weight loss
- ✓ Blurred vision

- ✓ Needing to wee all the time (especially at night)
- ✓ Wounds that won't heal
- ✓ Itching around the penis or vagina
- ✓ Repeated episodes of thrush (in women)

Prevention and Treatment

To avoid Type 2 diabetes, and also to stay healthy if you already have diabetes, eat healthily, take regular exercise and try to maintain a healthy weight. Also, drink alcohol in moderation and don't smoke.

The aim of treatment is to keep your blood glucose stable. This, together with a healthy lifestyle, will help to prevent complications. For Type 1 diabetes you need to use an insulin injection or pump – it is vital that this is used several times a day to keep blood glucose stable. For Type 2 diabetes, if a healthy lifestyle is not enough to control your symptoms, you may need to take tablets as well, but because Type 2 diabetes is progressive, you too may eventually need to start using self-administered injections or a pump, instead. It is important to look after your feet and have regular eye tests as people with diabetes are prone to problems with both.

Hypoglycaemic Attack

If someone has a hypoglycaemic attack (hypo) they may be shaky, sweaty, hungry, and/or have tingling lips, a pale face, heart palpitations (irregular heart beats), increased heart rate and feel confused and irritable. The first thing you should do is give them something sugary, such as a glass of fruit juice, sugar lumps, chocolate, glucose tablets or dextrose gel; then give them a longer-acting carbohydrate food such as a few biscuits, or a sandwich.

Hypothyroidism (Under-active Thyroid)

You'll find your thyroid gland at the base of your neck just below your voice box (larynx). It manufactures the hormones that control how fast our bodies work. If it makes too little we put on weight and feel lacking in energy. This sometimes happens because an autoimmune condition attacks the cells of the thyroid gland (autoimmune thyroiditis). Babies can also be born with an abnormal thyroid (congenital hypothyroidism). Hypothyroidism affects six times as many women as men. Hypothyroidism often comes on gradually, so you may not notice any symptoms at first, but they include:

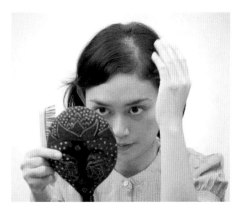

- Feeling tired and sleepy all the time
- Weight gain
- Dry, pale skin
- Muscle cramps and weakness
- Brittle nails
- Feeling cold all the time
- Coarse, thinning hair
- Hoarse, croaky voice
- Depression
- Erectile dysfunction in men

Prevention

In most cases, there is no way to prevent hypothyroidism. However, you do need some iodine in your diet for the thyroid gland to function properly. Good sources include:

- Iodized table salt (but don't have too much!)
- Milk and dairy products
- Fish and seafood

Treatment

Thyroxine replacement is used to treat hypothyroidism. This is taken in tablet form and replaces thyroxine, the hormone you lack. Your doctor will normally start you off on a low dose and then adjust it over a number of months until it's at the right level for you. You will have to take this medication for the rest of your life.

Hyperthyroidism (Over-active Thyroid)

Your thyroid gland controls how fast your body works. If it produces too much of the hormone thyroxine, your body goes into overdrive. You will feel restless, jittery and emotional and may start to lose weight. One common cause of hyperthyroidism is Graves' disease, in which antibodies stimulate the thyroid gland to produce too much thyroxine. Hyperthyroidism affects many more women than men. As with hypothyroidism, symptoms often come on gradually and may include:

- Feeling restless, emotional and irritable
- Hyperactivity
- Weight loss
- Difficulty sleeping
- Tremor in the hands

- Heart palpitations
- Shortness of breath
- Diarrhoea
- Swollen thyroid gland (goitre)
- Eye problems (if you have Graves' disease)

Prevention and Treatment

An important preventative measure is not to smoke (you are more likely to get Graves' disease if you smoke). Treatment includes:

- **Thionamides:** These drugs reduce the amount of thyroxine produced by your thyroid gland. They can make you prone to infections so tell your doctor immediately if you get a fever, sore throat or any other sign of infection.
- **Beta-blockers:** These can relieve some of the symptoms of hyperthyroidism, including heart palpitations.
- **Radio iodine:** This involves swallowing a capsule or taking a drink that contains radioactive iodine. This gathers in the thyroid gland and destroys some of the tissue that produces thyroxine. You will need to stay away from other people for a few weeks after the treatment.
- **Surgery:** Doctors will remove part of the thyroid gland.

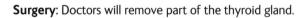

Sexual health

Looking after your sexual health is an important part of having an enjoyable sex life. Sexually transmitted infections are on the increase, and often don't have obvious symptoms. Unless you are in a committed monogamous relationship, making sure you always have safe sex – by using a condom, for example – is vital. If you do develop symptoms of any kind it's always a good idea to go and have them checked out at your local genito-urinary medicine (GUM) clinic.

Chlamydia

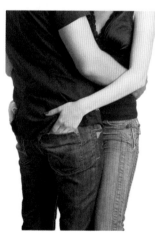

Chlamydia is a very common sexually transmitted infection caused by a bacterium called chlamydia trachomatis. You can pick it up during unprotected vaginal, anal or oral sex. Both men and women can catch it. Chlamydia is easy to diagnose and simple to treat, but because most people don't get any symptoms it often goes undetected. Many people are only diagnosed once they've had the infection for a while.

The problem with this is that, left untreated, chlamydia can cause serious complications. It can lead to a condition called pelvic inflammatory disease in women. This may damage the fallopian tubes that carry the egg from the ovaries to the womb and cause infertility. It can also harm men's fertility by causing inflammation in the testicles.

Symptoms

Lots of people have no symptoms to begin with and symptoms can take months, or even years, to appear. Women may notice:

- Pain on weeing
- A change in vaginal discharge
- Lower tummy pain
- Pain or bleeding during sex
- Bleeding between periods

Men may notice:
- Irritation on tip of penis
- Cloudy white discharge from the penis
- Pain on weeing
- Tenderness in the testicles

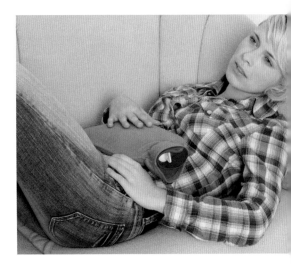

Prevention
- Use a condom whenever you have vaginal or anal sex
- Use a condom to cover the penis if you have oral sex, or a latex or plastic square (dam) to cover the female genitals
- Don't share sex toys, or carefully wash them and cover them with a new condom before using them with someone else

Treatment
Your doctor will take a swab or ask you for a urine sample to confirm that you have chlamydia before treating you. As chlamydia is a bacterial infection, a course of antibiotics is usually enough to clear it up. It may be a single dose (azithromycin) or a longer course lasting one week (doxycycline). Your partner, or partners, will need to take the treatment, too.

Did You Know?

Chlamydia can lead to a rare complication called reactive arthritis, particularly in men. This causes inflammation in the joints and needs treating with anti-inflammatory drugs, such as ibuprofen. Symptoms usually get better in three to 12 months, but can recur.

Genital warts

Genital warts are small pinkish-white lumps or larger cauliflower-shaped lumps on or around the genitals. They are caused by the human papilloma virus (HPV). They are spread by sexual contact and appear on or around the penis, vagina and anus. Warts on other parts of the body are caused by different strains of HPV so are rarely transmitted to the genitals. Some strains of the HPV virus are associated with an increased risk of cervical cancer.

Prevention

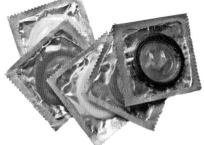

- There are vaccines available against the strains of HPV that are most likely to increase your risk of cervical cancer
- Use a condom whenever you have sex
- Use a condom to cover the penis if you have oral sex, or a latex square (dam) to cover the vulva
- Don't share sex toys, or carefully wash them and cover them with a new condom before using them again

Treatment

- **Podophyllin**: A brown liquid that is painted onto the warts by a doctor or nurse. You may need several applications.
- **Podophyllotoxin lotion or gel**: You can apply this at home. It takes up to four weeks to work.
- **Cryotherapy**: Your nurse or doctor will use liquid nitrogen to freeze off more persistent warts.
- **Electrocautery**: This involves using an electric needle to burn the warts off. You'll be given a local anaesthetic first.

Genital Herpes

Genital herpes is a very common sexually transmitted infection. It's caused by the herpes simplex virus, which also causes cold sores. Once you have caught the virus it stays in your body and causes further outbreaks. Most people have about four to five outbreaks in the first two years after being infected. The severity of the outbreaks usually decreases over time. People often don't get any symptoms when they first catch the virus and may be unaware that they have it.

Symptoms

Some people have no symptoms, but you may notice:

- 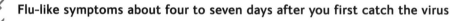 **Flu-like symptoms about four to seven days after you first catch the virus**
- **Painful red blisters on or around your genitals**
- **Vaginal discharge**
- **Pain on weeing**

Prevention

- **Use a condom whenever you have sex**
- **Use a condom to cover the penis if you have oral sex, or a latex square (dam) to cover the female genitals (these may not be easy to find, so you could try clingfilm)**
- **Don't share sex toys**

Treatment

If you are having your first outbreak of genital herpes, it's probably best to be treated at a genito-urinary medicine (GUM) clinic.

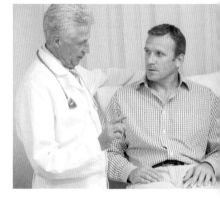

- **Acyclovir tablets**: These work by stopping the virus multiplying. They can prevent outbreaks or dampen them down once they have started.
- **Self help**: Taking a simple painkiller, such as paracetamol, will help to ease pain. You'll need to avoid sex while the virus is active, too.

Gonorrhoea

Gonorrhea is a bacterial infection spread by sexual contact. It can infect the cervix, urethra (the tube that carries urine from the bladder), back passage and throat. Gonorrhea is easily diagnosed and treated, but women may not know that they have it as the symptoms are vague. Like chlamydia, gonorrhea can cause other health problems, such as pelvic inflammatory disease, which may lead to infertility. You cannot get gonorrhea from kissing or sharing plates and cutlery.

Symptoms

Many women have no symptoms, but you may notice:

- **Strong-smelling, yellow-greenish vaginal discharge**
- **Pain or burning on weeing**
- **Irritation of, or discharge from, back passage**
- **Bleeding between periods**

Symptoms tend to be more obvious in men:

- **White or yellow discharge from the penis**
- **Pain or burning on weeing**
- **Tenderness in testicles**
- **Irritation of, or discharge from, back passage**

Prevention

- **Use a condom whenever you have sex**
- **Use a condom to cover the penis if you have oral sex, or a latex square (dam) to cover the female genitals**
- **Don't share sex toys, or carefully wash them and cover them with a new condom before using them again**

Treatment

Your doctor will take swabs to confirm your diagnosis before treating you. You'll be given a single dose in tablet or injection form. Your symptoms should clear within days. Your doctor will advise you not to have sex until the infection has definitely cleared. Your partner, or partners, will need to be treated, too.

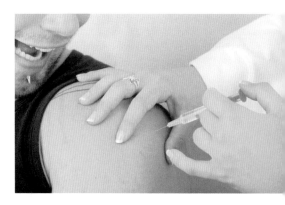

HIV and AIDS

Human immunodeficiency virus (HIV), spreads via bodily fluids and breast milk. It's usually caught during sexual contact. While most viruses attack cells in the body the HIV virus attacks the immune system. AIDS (auto immune deficiency syndrome) is the term used to describe the last stages of HIV infection where the immune system is so damaged that it can no longer fight off infections and diseases like cancer. Without treatment, it takes about 10 years for somebody who was previously healthy to get to this stage.

Symptoms

Some people get flu-like mild symptoms when they first catch the virus. Signs of AIDS may include:

 Opportunistic infections, such as pneumonia
AIDS-related cancers, such as non-Hodgkin's lymphoma

Prevention

Use a condom whenever you have sex
Use a condom to cover the penis if you have oral sex, or a latex square (dam) to cover the female genitals
Don't share sex toys, or carefully wash them and cover them with a new condom before using them again

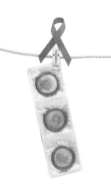

Treatment

Antiretroviral drugs are used to reduce levels of HIV in the body. This allows the immune system to recover so that it can work more effectively. Side effects can be severe, but your doctor will help you manage these. Antiretroviral drugs help many HIV-positive people to live long and healthy lives.

Checklist

- **Moisturize:** To keep your skin healthy, moisturize it regularly, particularly your hands which are vulnerable to contact dermatitis.
- **Dry your skin:** Always dry the skin thoroughly after showers, baths and swimming to avoid fungal infections.
- **Take the load off:** If you stand for long periods in the course of your job, take regular breaks to reduce your risk of varicose veins.
- **Be good to your heart!** That means a healthy diet, no smoking, not too much alcohol and regular exercise.
- **Blood pressure:** If you are over 50 get your blood pressure checked regularly to lower your risk of heart attacks and strokes.
- **Iron:** Get plenty of iron to prevent anaemia. Good sources include lean red meat, green leafy vegetables and fortified breakfast cereals.
- **Exercise for bones:** Do plenty of weight-bearing exercise, such as running and weight training, when you are young to lower your risk of osteoporosis. But only do it in moderation as you get older to ward off osteoarthritis.
- **Calcium for bones:** Eat lots of calcium-rich foods, such as dairy products and tinned sardines, to keep your bones healthy.
- **Safe sex:** If you are single, always use a condom when you have sex to keep yourself safe from sexually transmitted infections.

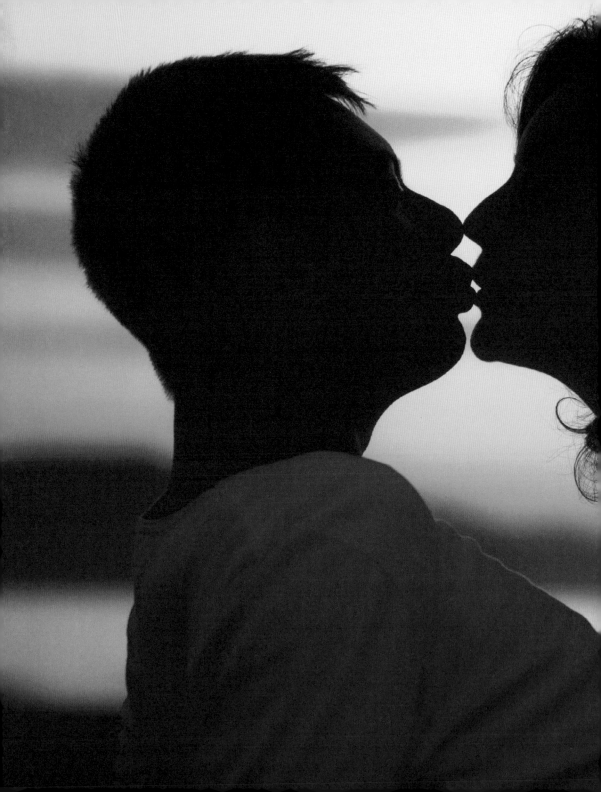

Men & Women's Health

Men's Health

Men have particular issues involving their fertility, sex organs, hormones, sexual performance, male pattern baldness and erectile dysfunction, plus prostate and testicular cancer. Generally men are more reluctant about getting help on health issues, preferring to ignore symptoms and it tends to be their partners who nag them to see a doctor.

Male Pattern Baldness (Androgenic Alopecia)

Men can suffer hair loss from as early as their teens, although it usually starts in the 20s and 30s. It affects almost two-thirds of men and by 60 most men will have experienced some hair loss. It's regarded as a natural part of ageing and not a disease.

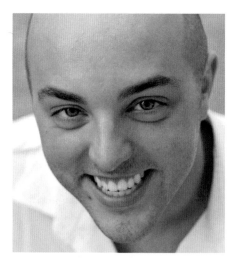

Symptoms
These include:

- A receding hairline
- Followed by thinning of the hair on the top of the head and temple
- Eventually these merge into a 'bald spot' leaving the remaining hair in a horseshoe shape

What Causes It?
It's all down to your genes. The male sex hormone testosterone produces dihydrotestosterone (DHT) and this causes the hair follicles to shrink to the extent that they eventually find it difficult to grow new hair.

Treatment

There is no cure but some treatments can slow down hair loss. These include:

- **Minoxidil (Regaine)**: This is a lotion that you apply to your scalp and in about 50 per cent of cases it will slow down hair loss; 15 per cent of men who use it may notice some new hair growth, but in one-third of cases it doesn't make any difference.
- **Finasteride (Propecia)**: This is a pill that blocks the effects of male hormones (anti-androgens). It's been shown to slow down hair loss and promote re-growth in 80 per cent of cases after three to six months.

Male Fertility

Fertility in men is judged on the quality and quantity of sperm in semen. One in six couples has problems conceiving and in about a third of cases there is some sort of male infertility factor.

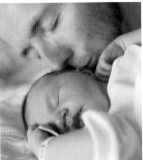

How is Fertility Measured?

If you and your partner are having infertility investigations, the doctors will ask you for a semen sample which will be analysed for:

- **Sperm count**: The normal range is 20 to 600 million sperms, per millilitre (ml), in a volume of 1 to 4 ml. A low sperm count is called oligozoospermia. It can be confusing though because you can have a normal sperm count and be sub fertile – for it also depends on the quality of the sperm.
- **Sperm motility**: This is the proportion of sperm which are moving – only those with rapid forward movement are considered viable. Low sperm motility is called asthenozoospermia.
- **Sperm morphology (shape)**: Up to 40 per cent of sperm may be abnormal in a fertile man's sperm – but problems arise when the majority of sperm are misshapen and defective. This condition is called teratozoospermia.
- **No sperm at all**: Some men do not produce any sperm and this is called azoospermia.

Did You Know?

It's a myth that abstinence makes sperm more potent – although more sperm may have built up, the quality will have deteriorated.

How to Boost Fertility

Fertility in men is affected by a number of factors (*see* below).

 Avoid wearing tight clothing: Think loose trousers and boxers rather than tight jeans and briefs. This is because sperm need to be cooler than body temperature to be in the best condition.

 Take a shower rather than a hot bath: Sperm need to stay cooler than body temperature – so no long hot soaks for you.

 Stop smoking and drinking: Both affect sperm quality.

 Take care with your diet: Zinc can boost fertility so consider a supplement or eating zinc-rich foods such as brazil nuts, eggs and seafood (*see* page 25). Include plenty of fresh fruit and vegetables too for their high vitamin C content.

 Keep in general good health: Even minor colds and coughs can affect sperm quality (production takes 73 days from start to finish).

 Don't smoke cannabis or take steroids for bodybuilding: Both can affect sperm quality.

 Lose weight: Fertility in overweight men may be affected by excess fat causing an increased temperature around the testes.

 Avoid chemicals: Some chemicals such as pesticides, flame retardants in furniture and substances used in food packaging etc. can block the male hormone androgen and lower sperm count.

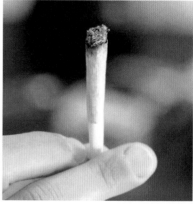

Treatment

Intra-Cytoplasmic Sperm injection (ICSI) is used as part of In Vitro Fertilization (IVF). It involves taking a single sperm from a man's sperm and injecting it in the partner's egg. ICSI is now used in 50 per cent of IVF cases and has revolutionized IVF care for men.

Prostate Health

The prostate gland is the size and shape of a walnut and is situated between your penis and bladder. It helps produce the fluid element of semen. The three main types of disease that affect the prostate all have similar symptoms and can be difficult to distinguish without investigations.

Benign Prostatic Hyperplasia (BPH)

This is a condition where the prostate becomes enlarged, most probably due to changes in hormone levels as you age, and is therefore experienced by middle-aged and elderly men. These men will often complain about having to get up to go to the loo at night or needing to pee more frequently. Other symptoms include reduced stream, hesitancy in starting to pee, urgency, dribbling and a feeling of not being able to empty your bladder properly. By the time you reach your 70s, you'll have a 75 per cent chance of suffering problems passing urine. Treatments include:

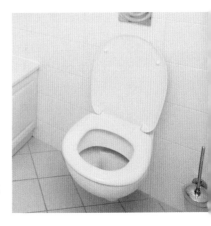

- **Self-help measures**: These include avoiding drinks containing caffeine (cola, tea and coffee) and not drinking close to bedtime, plus increasing your fibre intake to avoid constipation and putting pressure on the bladder.
- **Drugs**: Alpha-blockers can relax the muscle tone in your bladder making it easier to pee, and finasteride reduces the size of the prostate so urine can pass through more easily.
- **Surgery**: An operation to remove either part of or the whole prostate can be removed called a prostatectomy. However surgery can cause a number of long-term side effects such as 'dry' ejaculation (where semen is expelled back into the bladder) and incontinence.

Prostatitis

This is the medical name for inflammation of the prostate and can be acute – caused by a bacterial or viral infection, including sexually transmitted disease – or chronic, the cause of which is unclear. Treatments include ibuprofen or paracetamol for pain relief and antibiotics to treat infection for an average of four to six weeks.

Prostate Cancer

This is the most common cancer in men (responsible for one in four male cancer cases) and the chances of developing it increase as you get older. Most cases are diagnosed in men over 65. Some of the symptoms are similar to BPH, which reinforces the importance of seeking medical help if you develop any of them, such as:

- **Difficulty passing urine (slow or weak urine flow)**
- **Frequent need to pee (10 times a day or more) – and at night**
- **Problems starting to pass urine**
- **Dribbling urine**
- **Pain when passing urine or ejaculating (usually associated with prostatitis)**
- **Pain in the testicles or lower back**
- **If prostate cancer has not been diagnosed and has spread you may notice blood in the urine, bone and back pain and pain in the testicles**

For diagnosis, there are a number of investigations your doctor may carry out or arrange to be done, such as kidney function tests, tests for bacterial infections and an ultrasound scan of the bladder, as well as:

- **Digital rectal examination:** This is an examination of the prostate where a doctor inserts a gloved finger so they

Did You Know?

Prostate cancer is more common in Afro-Caribbean and African men. In 80 per cent of cases it is slow growing and develops over many years or it can be more aggressive and develop quite quickly.

can feel your prostate (although uncomfortable, this shouldn't hurt).

 Bladder and urethra examination: This is done by passing a (microscopic) camera through the penis into the bladder to get a view of the bladder and urethra.

 Blood test: This test will measure levels of a protein produced by the prostate gland called Prostate Specific Antigen (PSA). High levels can mean there is a problem with your prostate – it is either enlarged, inflamed or has developed cancer, but it's also possible to have raised PSA levels and not have a problem with the prostate, which is why other tests should be done as well. Newer tests may well become available in the near future.

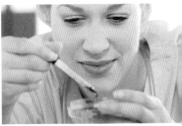

 Biopsy: A biopsy will be done if your doctor suspects your prostate is cancerous and involves removing a sample of tissue with a needle.

Prostate cancer can be treated and controlled effectively if caught early enough. There are a number of different treatments available:

 Watch and wait: If your cancer is slow growing and you have no symptoms (some cancers take 15 years to spread beyond the prostate) your doctor may decide to just closely monitor your prostate with regular blood tests and checkups.

 Surgery: *See* page 157.

Radiotherapy: This uses precisely-targeted high-energy rays to kill cancer cells.

Brachytherapy: A newer treatment used to treat early-stage prostate cancer, which uses radioactive seeds to more accurately target the cancer with less risk of damaging surrounding organs, reducing the risk of incontinence and sexual problems.

Hormone treatment: This can be used to help control the growth of your cancer cells if the case has spread beyond the prostate. They work by reducing levels of testosterone (the male sex hormone which prostate cancer feeds on).

Chemotherapy: This kills the cancer cells by interfering with cell division, causing damaged cells to self destruct. It is often used in conjunction with the above treatments if cancer has spread.

Impotence: Erectile Dysfunction (ED)

This is the medical name for experiencing problems getting and maintaining an erection for penetrative sexual intercourse. It's an extremely common condition affecting as many as 50 per cent of men over 40, but only around 20 per cent seek medical help because of embarrassment.

Physical Causes

In 75 per cent of cases there is a physical cause for impotence – usually involving blood supply to the penis. This is why it's so important you don't ignore symptoms, as they can be a sign of other problems – such as heart and blood vessel disease, diabetes, prostate problems and depression – which should be treated regardless of the ED. Impotence can be caused by:

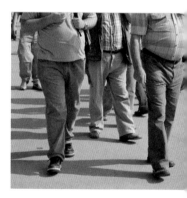

- High cholesterol and triglycerides (*see page 93*)
- Raised blood pressure
- Smoking, excess alcohol and drugs (recreational or prescribed)
- Diabetes
- Being overweight
- Stroke
- Prostate surgery
- Hormone imbalances
- Neurological diseases such as Parkinson's Disease and Multiple Sclerosis
- Nerve damage due to too much cycling (more than three hours a week) – hence why some saddles now have design features such as a groove up the middle

Psychological Causes

These can include:

- Stress: including work pressure and financial worries
- Marital discord

- Boredom with sexual partner
- Issues about sexual orientation
- Bereavement
- Anxiety about sexual performance

Treatment

Always see your doctor about ED problems as he will be able to run tests to check for more serious underlying problems, including heart disease.

- **Self–help measures**: Quitting smoking and cutting back on booze can all boost blood supply to your penis. Being physically fitter can also improve your circulatory system.
- **Check your medication**: ED or low libido can be a side effect of some drugs treatments including cholesterol-lowering statins, antidepressants and some high blood pressure drugs. Discuss your options with your doctor – do not simply stop the drugs.
- **Drug treatments**: There are a number of drugs available which can help you overcome ED; the three most well known are in a group called PDE5 inhibitors (sildenafil, tadalafil and vardenafil), which work by relaxing blood vessels in the penis encouraging blood to flow in and an erection to form. The effects (i.e. the *potential* to get an erection) last for several hours and you still need sexual stimulation. Also, the drug alprostadil can be administered as urethral suppositories and injections into the penis.
- **Manual treatments**: These include vacuum pumps which draw blood into the penis.
- **Other options**: These include surgery to increase blood flow and penile implants.
- **Psychological treatments**: These include counselling and talking therapies, such as cognitive behavioural therapies (*see* treatments for stress, page 42), sex therapy and so on.

Top Tip

Don't be tempted to order ED drugs from the internet, as, aside from quality concerns, you could miss out on a life–saving check–up. Research shows that *early* diagnosis of the underlying cause of ED could give you 2–3 years' warning of a potentially preventable heart attack.

Testicular Cancer

Ninety-five per cent of men make a full recovery from testicular cancer. Symptoms include a hard pea-sized (or larger) swelling or lump in the scrotum, a dull ache in the testicle or lower abdomen and a heavy feeling in the scrotum. If the cancer has spread, the man may find lumps in the collar bone or neck area or have a cough or breathing difficulties. Note: only one in 25 lumps will be cancerous – most are benign.

Causes

There are a number of risk factors, including:

- Having a father or brother with undescended testes
- Uncorrected undescended testes by age 11
- Complication of mumps

Did You Know?

If both testicles develop cancer, both of them will have to be removed. You will then need injections or patches of the male sex hormone testosterone to maintain your sex life. This is very unusual, however.

Diagnosis

- **Blood tests**: Checking for proteins produced by tumours.
- **Ultrasound**: Using sound waves, this gives doctors a picture of what is happening.
- **Biopsy (removal of one testicle)**: The 'biopsy' involves the actual removal of the testicle in order to reduce the risk of the cancer spreading, which would be increased by doing a normal biopsy. This doesn't affect your fertility or ability to have sex.
- **MRI scan, X-ray or CT scan**: This is to check the size and location of the tumour.

Treatment

- **Removal**: Surgical removal of the affected testicle.
- **Lymph node removal**: This only happens if the cancer is more advanced and has spread.
- **Chemotherapy**: If the cancer has spread you may need chemotherapy (see page 159). You'll be offered the chance to freeze sperm samples as the treatment risks infertility.
- **Radiotherapy**: (see page 159)

Hernia

A hernia is when an internal part of our body, such as tissue or one of our organs, pokes through the surrounding wall of muscle or tissue, causing a bulge. The most common type is an inguinal hernia, which appears in the groin. The lining of the gut, and often part of the gut itself, protrudes through a weakness in the abdominal wall, causing a lump at the site of the hernia, which may bulge with pressure, for example, when you cough. These nearly always affect men.

Sometimes a hernia can obstruct your bowel or the blood supply to part of the gut may be stopped (strangulated hernia). If you have intense pain, vomiting, redness or swelling seek medical help urgently.

Prevention

- ✅ Avoid lifting very heavy objects
- ✅ Don't smoke – a persistent cough due to smoking-related lung disease is associated with a higher risk of hernia

Treatment

You should always seek medical help for a hernia. Your doctor will probably suggest surgery (although unfortunately, in the UK, some primary care trusts will not fund routine hernia operations), during which the hernia is usually repaired using a special mesh to cover the hole in the abdominal wall. This may be done using open surgery – where the surgeon makes one large incision in your abdominal wall – or keyhole surgery. In keyhole surgery several small cuts are made and fine instruments passed through to carry out the procedure. Your doctor may suggest you wear an elasticated belt called a truss while you wait for surgery, but this is rarely done these days.

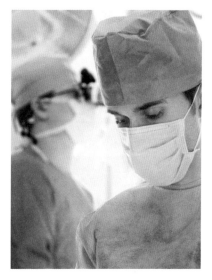

Women's Health

Like men, women have specific health problems connected with their sex organs, hormones and reproductive functions. Unlike men, women are usually better about seeking medical help for their problems earlier and more frequently.

Pre-Menstrual Syndrome (PMS)

Women begin their menstrual cycle at puberty (typically 10–14 years of age) and normally continue menstruating until the age of 50. Women's cycles last from 21 to 40 days with the average being 28 days. A number of medical conditions can affect the menstrual cycle and cause symptoms.

Pre-Menstrual Syndrome is the medical name for a range of physical and mental symptoms which happen in the two-week run-up to a period. Nine out of 10 women suffer some PMS symptoms. Forty per cent of women with PMS have distressing symptoms and five per cent say these symptoms are severe.

Symptoms
Symptoms vary considerably but can include:

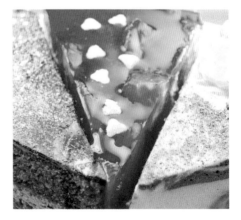

- Breast tenderness
- Depression
- Fatigue
- Cravings for carbohydrates, sweet or salty foods
- Irritability and mood swings
- Water retention and swollen ankles

Worsening of symptoms of other medical conditions such as asthma, allergies and epilepsy

 Acne or spots and other skin problems

Top Tip

Cut back on alcohol, salt and caffeine – all three can make PMS symptoms worse.

Natural Remedies

Lots of supplements and vitamin preparations are marketed to help alleviate PMS symptoms, but good scientific evidence is lacking for many of them.

 Agnus castus (chasteberry): This does have some clinical evidence to show that it relieves PMS symptoms. It works on the pituitary gland in the brain to balance production of the hormones progesterone and oestrogen, easing breast tenderness, tension, headaches and depression.

 Red Clover: This is another natural remedy believed to relieve PMS symptoms.

 Vitamin B6: May help the brain make serotonin (the 'feel good' brain chemical) and help alleviate depression associated with PMS, although there isn't much scientific evidence to support this.

 St John's Wort: This herbal remedy for depression can also bring relief and is backed by research. Note that this should not be used when taking a contraceptive pill. It has also been shown to interact with other drugs.

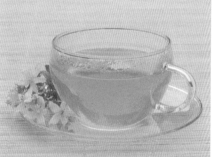

 Evening primrose: An essential fatty acid, this natural remedy was prescribed for breast tenderness, but more recent research suggests there is little scientific evidence to support its use, despite many patients feeling that it helps if enough is taken.

 Light therapy: There is some evidence that using light boxes' bright white light may ease depression and mood swings, but researchers are unsure of the mechanism.

Prescription Drugs

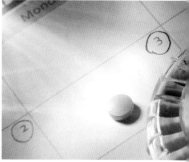

- ✔ **Antidepressants**: Drugs such as Prozac and other SSRIs (selective serotonin reuptake inhibitors) can help improve depression associated with PMS.
- ✔ **Combined oral contraceptive pills**: Some doctors prescribe the Pill for PMS. One type of combined pill in particular, Yasmin, has been shown to be beneficial.
- ✔ **Oestrogen patches**: The purpose of these is to suppress ovulation and therefore stop the monthly cycle which causes PMS.
- ✔ **Diuretics**: Reduce ankle swelling (but not abdominal bloating).
- ✔ **Mirena**: This Intra-Uterine System (IUS) is implanted into the womb and releases low doses of the hormone progestogen, reducing menstrual blood flow and some women report PMS symptoms improve too.
- ✔ **Male hormone treatments**: In severe cases treatment with a synthetic version of the male hormone testosterone may be considered as a treatment.

Surgery

In very severe cases of PMS and only when all other treatment options have been exhausted, doctors will consider performing an operation to remove the ovaries and a hysterectomy to remove the womb, but this is regarded as a last-resort option.

Did You Know?

The average modern woman can expect to have 450 periods in her lifetime compared with her ancestors who would only have had about 40 due to continual childbearing and lower life expectancy.

Heavy Menstrual Bleeding

This affects up to 20 per cent of women and is one of the most common reasons for having a hysterectomy. It's defined as losing more than 80 ml per period – but this is obviously very difficult to measure. It may help to keep a diary of your symptoms so you have a record of what is happening to you.

Symptoms

If you have more than two of the symptoms below you are suffering from heavy bleeding and should see your doctor for advice.

 Heavy blood flow (so severe you cannot leave the house for a couple of days)
Flooding that soils bed linen at night
Bleeding lasting eight to10 days
Passing blood clots other than in the first three days

Causes

Sometimes there is no obvious physical cause, but heavy bleeding can be a symptom of conditions such as fibroids, endometriosis (see page 170), pelvic inflammatory disease and endometrial cancer.

Drug and Hormone Treatment

There are a number of drug treatments your doctor can prescribe, which can help with heavy periods:

 Non steroidal anti-inflammatory drugs: Drugs such as ibuprofen and naproxen can reduce bleeding by inhibiting hormones called prostaglandins which are involved in menstrual blood blow. They also help block pain receptors in the muscle wall of the uterus.
 Tranexamic acid: This inhibits an enzyme which controls blood loss during menstruation and can reduce blood flow by 58 per cent.
Mirena IUS: This is a contraceptive implant but can also reduce blood flow by up to 80 per cent and some women have no periods at all. (See page 166.)
Contraceptive pill: The combination of the hormones oestrogen/progesterone in the Pill suppresses ovulation and thins the lining of the womb - so there is less blood loss during the artificial period that happens in the gap between pills. Some pills can be taken back-to-back without a break.

Male hormone treatments: Drugs using artificial versions of testosterone can be used to act on the ovary and thin the lining of the womb (endometrium). However side effects include acne and excess body hair growth.

 Other hormone treatments: There are a group of drugs called gonadotrophin-releasing hormone agonists (such as Zoladex) which induce a temporary menopause. However they have side effects including night sweats and hot flushes and affect bone density so are only prescribed as a short-term measure.

Surgical Treatment

There are a number of minimally invasive techniques available now to ease heavy bleeding as well as the more radical solutions such as hysterectomy (removal of the womb) and ovaries.

 Endometrial ablation: These use different energy sources (lasers, microwave etc.) to remove the lining of the womb to reduce menstrual blood flow. Most can be done under local anaesthetic on a day-case basis.

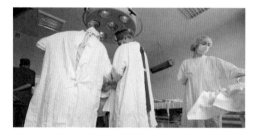

 Hysterectomy: Removal of the womb is only advised if other treatment options have failed, or you have condition such as cancer or a prolapse.

Did You Know?

Sixty per cent of women who see a gynaecologist for heavy bleeding will end up having a hysterectomy.

Polycystic Ovary Syndrome (PCOS)

This is the medical name for a range of symptoms associated with women developing tiny cysts on the ovaries. They contain egg follicles which have not developed properly due to hormonal difficulties. Women with PCOS produce higher than normal levels of the male hormone testosterone and it is this hormone which causes most of the symptoms.

Symptoms

- **Irregular or absent periods**: Most women with PCOS don't ovulate or only occasionally so periods can be absent or irregular.
- **Infertility problems**: You don't release eggs regularly so your chances of becoming pregnant are reduced.
- **Miscarriage**: PCOS carries an increased risk of this.
- **Excess body hair**: You may have unwanted facial or body hair.
- **Acne**: Spots on your face, back and neck can be a sign of PCOS.
- **Weight gain**: This is connected to developing insulin resistance where the body has to make larger amounts of insulin to control sugar levels and can cause weight gain, especially around the middle.

Diagnosis

PCOS is usually diagnosed through a combination of ultrasound and blood tests to check hormone and blood sugar levels. You may be referred to a gynaecologist.

Treatment

Whilst there is no cure for PCOS there are a number of treatments that can improve symptoms, including:

Did You Know?

PCOS puts women at higher risk of weight gain, heart disease, Type 2 diabetes and infertility.

- **Contraceptive pills**: The brands Dianette or Yasmin can improve acne and hirsuitism (excess body hair). (*See* page 166.)
- **Diabetes drugs**: Insulin resistance can be improved by drugs such as metformin (Glucophage).
- **Fertility drugs**: Clomiphene citrate can boost egg production.
- **Laparoscopy**: This is a type of surgery, involving the ovaries, that can help restore fertility.

Fibroids

These are non-cancerous growths in the womb. Around one in three women have fibroids, but most don't have symptoms. They're more common in overweight women, Afro-Caribbean women and women with no children or who had their last child at a young age.

Symptoms

- Heavy bleeding
- Pain (if the fibroids are large)
- Passing urine more frequently
- Constipation

Treatment

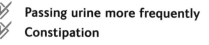

- **Uterine artery embolisation:** This blocks the blood supply to the fibroid causing it to shrink and can usually be performed under local anaesthetic.
- **Endometrial ablation:** (*See page 168.*)
- **Myomectomy:** This is an operation to remove the fibroid.
- **Hysterectom**y: (*See page 168.*)

Endometriosis

This involves the tissue normally lining the womb (endometrium) growing on different organs outside the womb, including the ovaries and an area behind the womb and in front of the rectum.

Symptoms

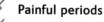

- Painful periods
- Painful sex
- Bloated feeling in lower abdomen

Treatment

Newer medications are undergoing trials, but currently treatment can include:

- NSAIDs (*see* page 167)
- Danazol
- Contraceptive pill
- Hysterectomy
- Laparoscopic surgery (to remove or destroy endometrial tissue)

Fertility and Conception

You can boost your chances of conceiving by giving up smoking, cutting down on alcohol, losing weight (if you're overweight) or gaining weight (if you're underweight) and eating a healthy, balanced diet and taking a 400 mcg folic acid supplement (*see* pages 23 and 29).

Fertile Times of The Month

Hormones trigger the release of an egg from your ovaries every month and a thickening of the lining of the womb for a fertilized egg to embed itself into. If you have a normal 28-day cycle your ovaries should release the egg on the 14th day (although cycles vary in length – in which case the date of ovulation is more tricky to predict). There is then just a 12–24-hour time period when it's possible to become pregnant. Doctors advise having regular sex and not getting too hung up about 'fertile' days.

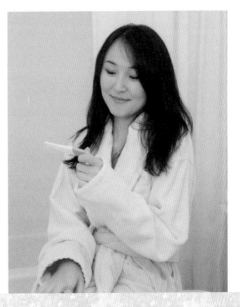

What Happens After an Egg is Fertilized?

If an egg is fertilized by sperm it will attach itself to the lining of the womb and multiply from a single cell to an embryo. Pregnancy can be detected by testing for the presence of hormones in a urine test a couple of days after a missed period.

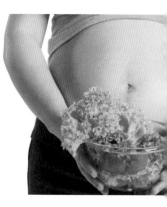

What Happens In Pregnancy?

In the first few weeks you may experience breast tenderness, nausea, tiredness, constipation, fatigue, increased frequency in peeing or a metallic taste in your mouth.

What Are The Stages of Pregnancy?

Pregnancy lasts for 40 weeks (pregnancy is dated from the first day of your last period), which is split into three trimesters:

- **First trimester (the first 12 weeks)**: By eight weeks the foetus is the size of a strawberry and by 12 weeks measures around 8 cm/3 inches. All the systems in the body are formed by 12 weeks. In the remainder of the pregnancy, organs and systems grow and mature.
- **Second trimester (12–24 weeks)**: By 17 weeks your baby has grown to 14 cm/5½ inches and by 18 weeks sex organs can be detected by scan. You may be feeling a rush of pregnancy hormones and experience a 'bloom'. By 20 weeks you should be able to feel your baby moving.
- **Third trimester**: Your baby is growing and maturing preparing for birth. You should have gained 11 kg/25 lb to 14 kg/30 lb and as your due date approaches your cervix will soften and your baby move into a head-down position ready for birth.

Eating in pregnancy

You don't need to eat for two in pregnancy – just an extra 200 calories a day in the last trimester (about two slices of toast!).

Did You Know?

Only five per cent of babies arrive on their estimated delivery date, but 80 per cent are born within 10 days of it.

Take a 400 mcg folic acid supplement for the first three months (*see* tip box on page 29), and there are certain foods you should avoid or limit:

- **Avoid mould-ripened cheeses**: Camembert, Danish Blue, Brie etc. should be avoided – this is because of the risk that they may be contaminated with listeria, a type of bacteria which can harm you and your baby. Hard cheeses and cottage cheese are fine though.
- **Cut out pâté**: Meat and vegetable pâtés may also be contaminated with listeria; meat pâtés may also contain high concentrations of Vitamin A – which can be harmful to the development of eyesight in the foetus.
- **Think about peanuts**: Some pregnant women choose to avoid peanuts if they have a history of allergies in the immediate family such as asthma and eczema but there is little scientific evidence that eating peanuts will increase the likelihood of your baby developing a peanut allergy.
- **Limit your caffeine intake**: Do not have more than 200 mg a day. Caffeine is found in coffee, tea, cola and chocolate and can cause your baby to have a low birth weight and may increase risk of miscarriage if consumed in large quantities. A mug of instant coffee contains 100 mg, a mug of filter coffee 140 mg, a cup of tea 75 mg, a can of cola 40 mg and a 50g bar of chocolate 50 mg.
- **Limit oily fish**: Eat no more than two portions of oily fish (mackerel, herring, trout) a week. Avoid shark, marlin and swordfish completely because of the risk of mercury contamination which can affect your baby's nervous system development.
- **Cut out alcohol**: Or at least drink no more than one or two units of alcohol once or twice a week.

Top Tip

Cook eggs until the yolk and white are solid. There is a risk of contracting salmonella, a type of food poisoning, from raw or undercooked eggs. Avoid products made with raw eggs such as mayonnaise and chocolate mousse.

Coping With Pregnancy Health Niggles

- **Ease pregnancy nausea**: Early in pregnancy your body is flooded with hormones which can make you nauseous. Try nibbling ginger biscuits, sipping ginger beer, or acupressure bands.

Avoid constipation: When you're pregnant your body produces more of a hormone that relaxes muscle tone and this slows down digestion. Drink plenty of water to soften your stools and eat high-fibre foods including whole grains and fruit and vegetables.

 Beat insomnia: It can be uncomfortable sleeping and you may find you're restless. Add lavender oil to your bath water and have a milky drink at bedtime to help you relax.

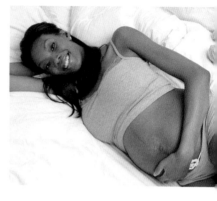

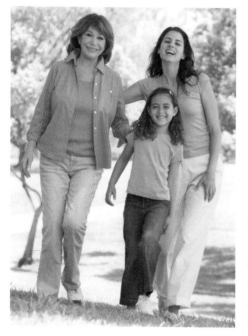

Menopause

Menopause refers to the end of menstruation (periods). You have reached the menopause if your periods have stopped for at least a year. The average age of menopause is 52. Menopausal symptoms can last two to five years, although some women suffer them for much longer.

Symptoms

Eight out of 10 women experience menopause symptoms and around 45 per cent will find their symptoms difficult to cope with. They are caused by the sudden fall in levels of the hormone oestrogen. Symptoms include:

 Hot flushes
Night sweats
Vaginal dryness

 Mood swings
Depression

Diagnosis

A blood test to measure levels of Follicle Stimulating Hormone (FSH) may give some indication of whether you are menopausal but is not definitive.

Top Tip

Natural remedies that might ease menopausal symptoms include sage, black cohosh and red clover, but there is no definite medical evidence of their efficacy.

Treatment

Hormone replacement therapy (HRT), in the form of pills and patches, can help alleviate the symptoms of the menopause including hot flushes and mood swings. However there are number of health risks attached to HRT so it's worth weighing them up before you decide to go ahead. They include a higher risk of breast, ovarian and womb cancer, blood clots and coronary heart disease and stroke. On the positive side it's an effective treatment, which helps prevent osteoporosis and reduces the risk of cancer of the colon and rectum.

Cervical Cancer

There are three main types of gynaecological cancers: cancer of the cervix, ovarian cancer and cancer of the womb (endometrial cancer). Cervical cancer is the second most common cancer in women aged under 35. It affects the neck of the womb. Some countries – including the UK – have a national screening programme to carry out smear tests every three years. It can be successfully treated in the early stages.

Causes

Over 99 per cent of cases are caused by the human papilloma virus (HPV). Many countries have now introduced vaccination programmes for teenage girls to protect women from developing cervical cancer in the future.

Symptoms

Cervical cancer doesn't always have symptoms, which is why attending screening appointments is important. However some women experience abnormal bleeding, after sex for example.

Treatment

 Early stage cancer: This can be treated with surgery. Options include a cone biopsy where a cone-shaped piece of the cervix is removed, or radical trachlectomy, where the cancer is removed but the internal opening of the cervix is stitched leaving a small opening. You may also be offered radiotherapy.

Later stage cancer: Hysterectomy (*see* page 168) and/or chemotherapy and radiotherapy will be offered.

Ovarian Cancer

Ovarian cancer affects women of all ages but is much more common in women over 50. In the past this was known as the 'silent killer' as it didn't appear to have any symptoms, but newer research suggests it does have early warning signs.

Symptoms

Bloating

Difficulty eating and feeling full more quickly than you used to

Abdominal and pelvic pain

Diagnosis

The outcome of treatment is much better if you are diagnosed early but unfortunately the majority of women are not being diagnosed until a later stage. Ovarian cancer is usually diagnosed through a combination of the following tests:

Blood test for the CA125 protein produced by some ovarian cancers (does not always indicate cancer)

Internal examination

Ultrasound

CT scan

MRI scan

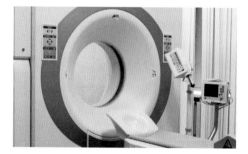

Treatment

This will depend on the stage the cancer has reached, but includes removal of the ovaries, hysterectomy and/or chemotherapy and radiotherapy.

Endometrial Cancer

This type of cancer affects the lining of the womb and is associated with older women (75 per cent of cases are in post-menopausal women). It is also associated with obesity. Treatment options include hysterectomy and radiotherapy/chemotherapy.

Symptoms

- ✅ Any bleeding in post-menopausal women
- ✅ Heavier bleeding in women who haven't gone through the menopause
- ✅ Pain during sex
- ✅ Pain in the lower abdomen

Did You Know?

Only one in 10 cases of unusual vaginal bleeding is caused by cancer.

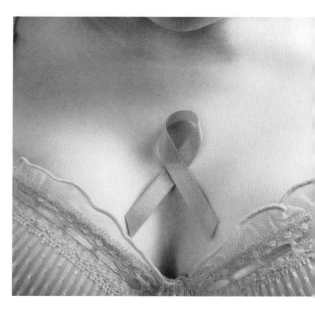

Breast cancer

Breast cancer is the most common cancer in women and mainly affects women over 40. Most countries now have mammogram (x-ray of the breasts) screening programmes and because of this and improvements in treatments, breast cancer is now highly treatable with a 10-year survival rate of 88 per cent if it is diagnosed and treated in the early stages after being detected by screening.

Symptoms

Always check your breasts monthly (a few days after your period is a good time as your breasts are less tender) for signs of any of the following:

- Lump or thickening in an area of the breast (remember that nine out of ten lumps are benign)
- Change in shape or size of the breast
- Dimpling of the skin
- Change of nipple shape
- Blood-stained discharge from the nipple
- Rash on a nipple or surrounding area
- Lump or swelling in your armpit

Diagnosis

Investigations include breast examination and ultrasound. A biopsy may also be taken; this is where a small sample of cells is taken from your breast using a needle and then examined under a microscope to see if they are cancerous.

Treatment

Treatment will depend on the stage your cancer has reached:

- **Lumpectomy**: Removal of the lump only may be possible if there is no evidence of the cancer spreading to lymph nodes.
- **Mastectomy**: Removal of the breast and lymph nodes. This is done if your cancer is more advanced. You should be offered breast reconstruction.
- **Radiotherapy**: This is sometimes offered in conjunction with surgery to kill off any remaining cancer cells. (See page 159.)
- **Chemotherapy**: (See page 159.)
- **Tamoxifen**: This is a hormone treatment given to women who have a type of breast cancer cells with oestrogen receptors. It is used after surgery for early breast cancer for

five years. It can also be used before surgery to shrink a large tumour.

- **Aromatase inhibitors**: Some women are switched onto these drugs after being treated with Tamoxifen.

Checklist

- **Male fertility**: Men can boost fertility by quitting smoking and drinking and losing weight. Zinc-rich food may help too.
- **Testicular cancer**: Men should always check their testicles for signs of lumps.
- **Erectile dysfunction**: Seek help for ED as it could be an early warning sign of heart problems or diabetes.
- **Prostate health**: Men should get a blood test to check for raised PSA levels if they have problems urinating.
- **Eating in pregnancy**: Pregnant women should avoid certain foods, including pâté, mould-ripened cheeses and alcohol.

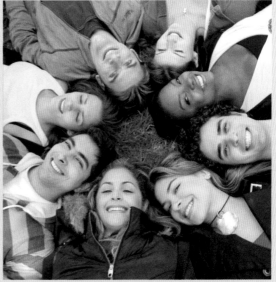

- **Vaginal and cervical health**: Any unusual vaginal bleeding should be checked out. Women need cervical smear tests to check for cervical cancer.
- **Breast health**: Women should check their breasts for abnormalities and older women aged over 50 should attend regular mammograms.

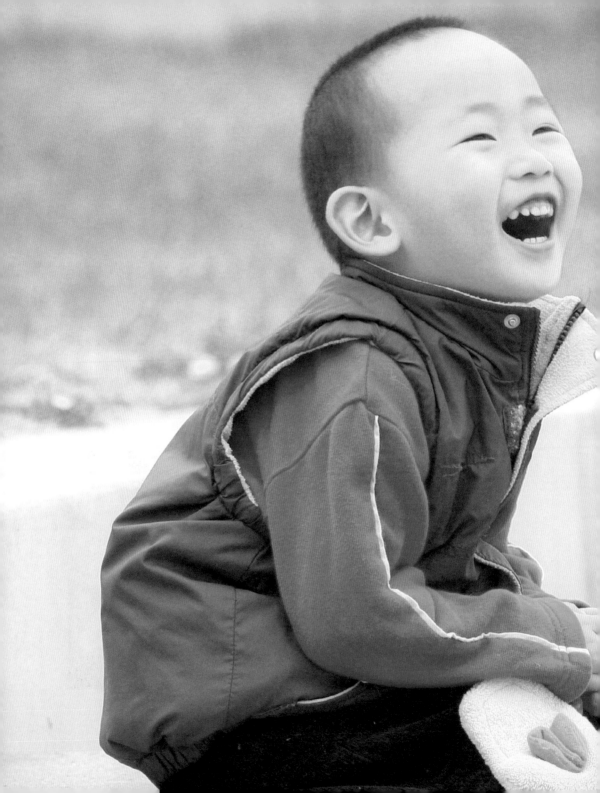

Children's Health

Ailments in Babyhood

One thing's for sure – at some point your baby *will* develop an ailment of some kind. That's because their immune system isn't fully mature yet, so they're more susceptible to bacteria and viruses than an adult. Most baby illnesses aren't serious, but it's still a good idea to have your baby checked out by a doctor if you have any concerns about their health.

Colic

All babies cry, but if your baby's crying is particularly inconsolable they may have colic. Colic is defined as repeated episodes of persistent crying in a baby who is otherwise fit and healthy. It's very common – about 20 per cent of babies have it – and it usually starts within a few weeks of birth. Although colic can be distressing for baby and parents alike, it isn't harmful and usually goes away on its own by the time your baby is four months old.

Symptoms

Colic symptoms are often worse in the evening. Your baby may:

- Cry furiously and inconsolably
- Go red and flushed in the face
- Arch their back, clench their fists and pull their knees up towards their tummy as though in pain
- Pass wind

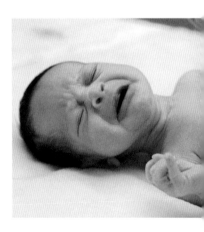

Prevention

- **If you are breastfeeding:** Avoid caffeine, alcohol and foods such as cauliflower and cabbage, that may give your baby wind.

If you are bottle-feeding: Check that the hole in the teat is not too small and causing them to swallow airas they feed.

 Burping: Always burp your baby after they feed.

Avoid over stimulation: Try not to over stimulate your baby by constantly picking them up and putting them down.

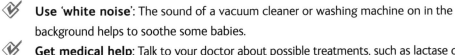

Top Tip

If your baby is bottle-fed, try holding him upright against your body as he feeds. This may help prevent him swallowing air along with his milk.

Treatment

Hold your baby: Cuddling your baby as he cries, or swaddling him in a sheet or thin cotton blanket, may help. However, if the crying becomes intolerable, it may be best to lay your baby safely in another room for a few minutes while you make yourself a cuppa or phone a friend for a good moan.

Try movement: Most babies find movement soothing. Gently rock your baby, take him for a walk in his pram or even for a drive in the car.

Use 'white noise': The sound of a vacuum cleaner or washing machine on in the background helps to soothe some babies.

Get medical help: Talk to your doctor about possible treatments, such as lactase drops.

Try an alternative therapy: Some parents find cranial osteopathy or massage helpful for colic. Do see a practitioner who is experienced in working with young babies.

Trust your instincts: If your baby has other symptoms, such as a rash or a fever, or if you just think something 'isn't quite right', don't hesitate to see your doctor.

Jaundice

Jaundice is a yellowish tinge to the skin and whites of the eyes. About 90 per cent of babies develop jaundice shortly after birth. It's caused by a yellow substance called bilirubin found in red blood cells. Newborns have extra red blood cells and sometimes become jaundiced when these are broken down. Jaundice isn't usually harmful, and should clear up on its own within a couple of weeks.

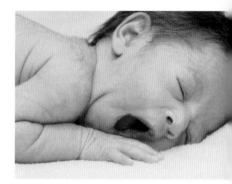

Symptoms

 Yellowish tinge to skin and whites of the eyes

 Your baby may be quite sleepy

Prevention and Treatment

Unfortunately, jaundice in newborns can't be prevented and most babies with jaundice don't need treatment. But if your baby's bilirubin levels are particularly high, or if the jaundice doesn't clear up within 10 to 14 days, there is a small risk of brain damage. In this case, your doctor may recommend:

 Treatment with UV light (phototherapy): For this, your baby will be placed naked except for an eye mask in a cot under a blue UV light for a few days. The UV light helps to break down the bilirubin.

 Feeding your baby often: This makes your baby produce more urine, which means the bilirubin is cleared from their body faster.

 Putting your baby in sunlight: Sunlight contains UV light, and so helps to break down the bilirubin. Never expose your baby to strong sunlight in the middle of the day. Morning or evening sun, or partial shade, is fine.

Fever

If your baby's temperature rises to 38°C (101°F) or more they have a fever. It can be worrying when your baby develops a fever, but take comfort in the fact that most ailments that cause fever in babies aren't serious. If they are still feeding and cheerful, they'll probably need nothing more than plenty of fluids and some extra cuddles.

Symptoms

If your baby becomes dehydrated, in addition to a temperature of 38°C (101°F) or above, you may notice:

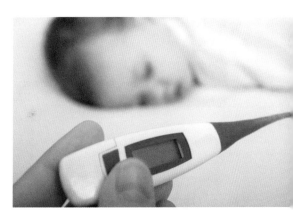

- Sunken eyes and fontanelles (the soft spots on your baby's head)
- Dry mouth
- Fewer wet nappies
- No tears when your baby cries

Prevention

- Don't let people who are obviously ill hold or kiss your baby
- Wash your hands regularly with soap and water
- Practise good hygiene when making up bottles and meals

Treatment

- **Plenty of fluids**: Offer your baby lots of drinks and milk feeds.
- **Baby paracetamol or ibuprofen**: If your baby is miserable, these anti-fever drugs should help him feel more comfortable.
- **Night-time checks**: Experts recommend checking your baby now and again during the night to make sure their condition hasn't worsened.
- **See your doctor if**: your baby is less than three months old; they develop a rash that doesn't disappear when pressed with a glass; they have a fit (convulsion) or if the fever lasts longer than 48 hours.

Top Tip

Sponging your baby down with tepid water may help to soothe and relax your feverish baby, but there is no evidence that it will help to bring the fever down. It is, however, recommended by most health-care professionals.

Colds

Believe it or not your baby may get up to 10 colds during their first year. That's because his immune system isn't mature yet, so he can't fight off cold viruses in the same way as you do. Most colds last about five to seven days and there's plenty you can do to keep him comfortable till he's better.

Symptoms

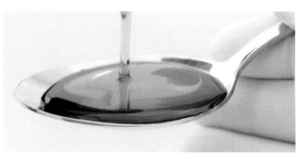

- Fever
- Cough
- Stuffed up, runny nose
- Irritability
- Loss of appetite

Prevention

Obviously you can't keep your baby wrapped in cotton wool, and it is important to remember that depsite all the potential dangers open to them, the vast majority of western-born babies fight off illness and go on to be strong and healthy individuals. But you can take some sensible precautions:

- Don't let anyone who has a cold near your baby
- Encourage the whole family to wash their hands regularly with soap and water
- Avoid crowded places
- Make sure your baby is well wrapped up when you go out in cold weather

Treatment

- **Offer plenty of fluids**: This will help keep your baby hydrated if they have a fever.
- **Try saline drops**: Saline nose drops (available from chemists) can help to clear your baby's nose before a feed. Only use nasal decongestants on your doctor's advice.
- **Consider anti-fever drugs**: If your child is miserable with a fever, baby paracetamol or ibuprofen can help.

✔ **See your doctor**: If your baby's breathing becomes rapid and shallow, they could have bronchiolitis. This is a potentially serious lung condition that requires medical attention.

Cradle Cap

Cradle cap is the common name for the greasy yellow scaly patches that sometimes appear on young babies' heads. It usually develops a few weeks or months after birth and clears up by the time a child is two. No one really knows what causes cradle cap, but some experts think it may be due to overactive sebaceous glands in babies' skin.

Symptoms

✔ **Greasy yellow patches on your baby's scalp**

✔ **Redness on the affected skin**

✔ **Patches may spread behind the ears and possibly to other parts of the body, such as the nappy area**

Did You Know?

Babies who get cradle cap often have a family history of allergies or allergic diseases, such as asthma or eczema.

Prevention and Treatment

Cradle cap can't be prevented and will eventually clear up on its own, but the following may help it on its way:

✔ **Apply oil**: Massage a little baby oil or petroleum jelly onto your baby's scalp and leave it overnight. In the morning brush your baby's hair or gently wipe their scalp with a flannel to remove any loose particles.

✔ **Shampoo regularly**: Washing your baby's hair once or twice a week with a mild baby shampoo may help to loosen the scales.

✔ **Look out for infection**: Occasionally, affected skin can become inflamed or infected. If you notice sore, red or irritated skin on your baby's scalp, or if the cradle cap starts to spread to other parts of the body, see your doctor.

Teething

Your baby will probably cut their first tooth around six to nine months. It's usually one of the bottom front teeth that comes through first. While some babies cut their teeth with barely a whimper, others have to endure days, or even weeks, of red-cheeked, drooling misery. Luckily, there are ways to ease the discomfort.

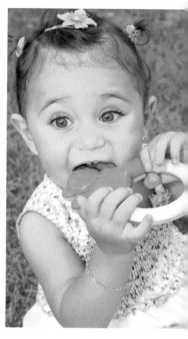

Symptoms

- **Chewing on fingers and toys**
- **Reddened cheeks**
- **Reddened gums**
- **Lots of dribbling**
- **Poor appetite because of painful gums**
- **Crying and irritability**

Prevention and Treatment

Sadly, little can be done to prevent the symptoms of teething before they begin, but the following treatments may help once teething starts:

- **Rub your baby's gums**: Gentle pressure with a clean finger may ease any discomfort.
- **Baby painkillers**: Baby paracetamol or ibuprofen administered at the recommended interval and dosage can help to ease teething pain.
- **Lots of cuddles**: Babies often find teething distressing. Soothing words and cuddles will help to reassure your baby.
- **Teething gels and granules**: Some parents find teething gels or homeopathic teething granules helpful, although there is no scientific evidence to support this.

Did You Know?

Children normally have a full set of baby teeth by the time they are two and a half to three years old.

Chilled teethers: Keep teething toys in the fridge for your baby to chew on when his gums are sore. Small sips of cold water may help, too.

Gastroenteritis (Diarrhoea and Vomiting)

Most babies have at least one bout of gastroenteritis before their first birthday. In babies it's usually caused by a virus called the rotavirus, and is often accompanied by a fever (see page 184). Most cases pass within a few days. The main risk to your baby is dehydration, so it's very important to offer them plenty of fluids.

Symptoms

 Vomiting and diarrhoea that come on rapidly
 Fever
 Tummy ache (*see* colic symptoms, page 182)
 Lack of appetite

If your baby becomes dehydrated, you may also notice:

 Dry mouth
 Sunken eyes and fontanelles (the soft patches on your baby's head)
 Fewer wet nappies than usual
 No tears when your baby cries

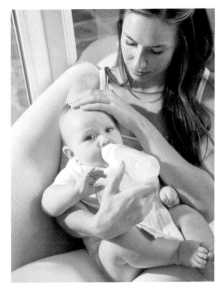

Prevention

Always wash your hands with soap and warm water after going to the toilet and changing nappies. Make sure other family members do the same. In the kitchen, wash your hands before and after preparing food and bottles, and keep surfaces and utensils spotlessly clean.

Treatment

As long as you give your baby plenty of fluids, they should start to be on the mend within a couple of days. If your baby hasn't improved within 48 hours, see your doctor. They may suggest oral rehydration solution (ORS). This comes as sachets of powder, which you add to water. It replaces salt, glucose and other minerals lost through dehydration.

Eczema

About 60 per cent of children who have eczema get it before their first birthday. The most common kind of eczema is atopic eczema, which runs in families along with other allergy-related conditions like hay fever and asthma. Atopic eczema tends to flare up now and again, but even between flare-ups the skin can be dry and itchy.

Symptoms

Eczema presents as itchy, red, dry skin that, in babies, often starts on the cheeks then spreads down to the neck and nappy area.

Prevention

- **Fish**: Some research suggests that including fish in your baby's weaning diet may protect against eczema.
- **Pre- and probiotics**: Other studies suggest that taking pre- and probiotics (supplements that promote the growth of 'friendly' bacteria in the gut) during pregnancy may reduce your baby's risk of eczema.

Top Tip

Applying emollients to your baby's still-wet skin after a bath significantly boosts their moisturizing effects. You may need to experiment with different emollients to find one that suits your baby.

Treatment

- ☑ **Avoid synthetic fibres and wool**: Use cotton bedding and clothing, instead.
- ☑ **Keep your baby's nails short**: This will help prevent damaged skin if he scratches.
- ☑ **Avoid triggers**: Soap, detergent, house dust mites and animal dander (dead skin scales) can all trigger eczema so keep them to a minimum.
- ☑ **Emollients**: Creams and bath oils recommended by your doctor can help keep dry skin moisturized and healthy. Use them frequently during flare-ups and then, when the eczema settles down, reduce use to once or twice a day.
- ☑ **Topical corticosteroids**: Used under your doctor's supervision, these are an effective way to reduce itching and inflammation.

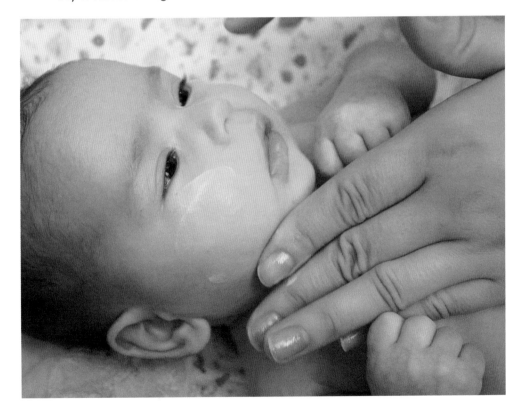

Nappy Rash

Nappy rash – a red, spotty rash that affects the nappy area – is very common in babies. It's caused by contact with urine and faeces and, although most cases are mild, it can be quite sore and persistent in some babies. Sometimes nappy rash is caused by an underlying condition, such as eczema or a fungal infection.

Symptoms

- Red or pink spots or blotches in your baby's nappy area
- Stinging when your baby wees or poos, or when you put them in the bath
- In serious cases, broken or infected skin

Top Tip

Don't use talcum powder on your baby's bottom. It won't protect their skin from urine and faeces, and may even irritate it more.

Prevention

- Change your baby's nappy regularly
- Apply a barrier cream to the nappy area at each change

Treatment

- **Let your baby's skin breathe**: Leave their nappy off from time to time so that the air can get to their skin.
- **Avoid irritants**: Soap and bath additives may aggravate the problem. Stick to water only until the rash clears up.
- **Try different nappies**: If you are using reusables try disposables and vice versa. Or try a different brand.
- **Be gentle**: Pat your baby's bottom dry instead of rubbing it.
- **For severe nappy rash**: See your doctor, who can prescribe a cream to help clear it up. Clotrimazole is often used – which will be familiar to many mums as a treatment for vaginal thrush – and is available without a prescription.

Childhood

By the time your child emerges from babyhood, their immune system will have matured and they will be able to fight off infections more easily. This is just as well because, when they go off to nursery, their immune system will be bombarded with all sorts of bugs, from head lice to chickenpox. Making sure your child eats well, exercises and gets plenty of sleep will help to keep them healthy and thriving throughout their school days.

Allergies

Allergies happen when your immune system overreacts to a substance that is normally harmless. A predisposition to allergies, known as atopy, tends to run in families. Common causes of childhood allergies are pollens, pets and house dust mites, as well as foods like nuts, eggs and fish. Allergic reactions can range from mild to extreme. Symptoms include:

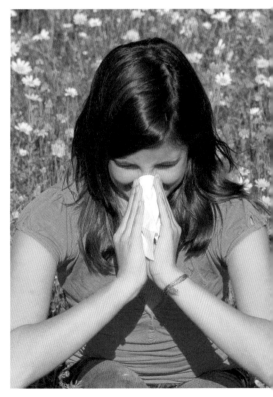

- ☑ **Swollen watery eyes**
- ☑ **Runny nose and sneezing**
- ☑ **Breathing difficulties**
- ☑ **Swollen, itchy face (angio-odema)**
- ☑ **Itchy rash (hives)**

If your child has a food allergy, they may also have:
- ☑ **Swollen, itchy mouth, tongue and lips**
- ☑ **Abdominal pain**
- ☑ **Nausea, vomiting or diarrhoea**

In severe cases, an extreme allergic reaction called anaphylaxis can occur. In this case, your child may experience:

- **Difficulty in speaking or swallowing**
- **Flushed skin**
- **Racing heart**
- **Feelings of weakness**
- **Unconsciousness**

Prevention

If you have a family history of allergies or atopic conditions like asthma and hay fever:

- **Don't eat peanuts while you are pregnant or breastfeeding**

- **Breastfeed exclusively for the first six months of your baby's life**
- **Don't smoke in front of your child**
- **Control the level of house dust mites in your home**

- **Don't keep pets, or restrict their access to parts of the house that your child regularly uses**

Treatment

Before treating your child, your doctor will carry out tests to find the cause of their allergies. Possible treatments include:

- **Avoidance:** Avoiding the allergy trigger or triggers is always the first step in treating allergies.
- **Antihistamines:** These can help with itching. They can be taken in tablet, cream and liquid form, or as drops.
- **Emollients:** These moisturizing creams and bath additives will soothe dry, itchy skin.
- **Steroids:** Steroid creams and inhalers can relieve swelling and inflammation on the skin and in the airways.

Adrenaline: Usually administered via a self-use injection, adrenaline rapidly reverses the symptoms of a severe allergic reaction. It is only available in the UK with a prescription, and if you have one on stand-by, keep an eye on the expiry date as it has a short shelf life.

Hyposensitization: This can help with a specific allergy to something like bee stings. Your child will gradually be introduced to more and more of the allergen to encourage their body to make antibodies that will stop future reactions.

Did You Know?

Some studies have shown a possible link between overuse of antibiotics in babyhood and a higher risk of childhood allergies. In any case, antibiotics should not be used excessively.

Chickenpox

Just about all children catch chickenpox at some point. It's caused by a highly infectious virus called the varicella-zoster virus. Your child will normally develop symptoms about 10 to 21 days after coming into contact with it. The virus stays in the body and may reactivate later in life as shingles. Luckily, for most children, it is a mild disease. The main symptom of an itchy red rash of spots (which turn into fluid-filled blisters with red rings around them) can be accompanied by:

 Fever　　 **Aches and pains**

Nausea　　**Loss of appetite**

Prevention and Treatment

Make sure all family members wash their hands regularly with soap and warm water and avoid places where you know the virus is active, such as your local parent and toddler group. If they do contract chickenpox, to keep your child comfortable and stop the virus spreading:

- **Keep them at home:** Your child shouldn't come into contact with other children until all their spots have crusted over. This will take about five to seven days. Also avoid pregnant women, as chickenpox can be harmful to unborn babies.
- **Calamine lotion:** Dabbing a little calamine lotion onto their spots will help to soothe the itching.
- **Cut their nails short:** This will help prevent scarring and infection if your child scratches their spots.
- **Offer children's paracetamol or ibuprofen:** Both can help to ease any fever or aches and pains.
- **Give them plenty of drinks:** Extra fluids will stop them getting dehydrated.
- **Homeopathy:** Homeopaths recommend the remedy pulsatilla if your child has chickenpox and is weepy, clingy and not thirsty, despite having a fever. Do consult a homeopath who is experienced in treating children before giving your child any remedies.

Measles

Measles is far less common than it used to be thanks to the MMR vaccination. But clusters of cases do still crop up from time to time, so it's wise to be aware of the symptoms. Measles is usually an uncomplicated disease, but in rare cases it can have potentially dangerous side effects, such as inflammation of the brain. Symptoms include:

- **Fever**
- **Dry cough**
- **Runny nose**

- Red, watery eyes
- Light sensitivity
- Red-brown rash that often starts behind the ears
- Small white spots in the mouth (Koplik's spots)

Prevention and Treatment

The most effective way to protect your child against measles is with the MMR vaccination. This also protects against mumps and rubella. To treat measles:

- **Offer children's paracetamol or ibuprofen**: Both can help to ease fever or aches and pains.
- **Give them plenty of fluids**: Children with measles can have quite a high fever, which may cause dehydration.
- **Plenty of rest**: Your child is likely to feel tired anyway.
- **Close the curtains**: This will help light-sensitive eyes.
- **Bathe their eyes**: Wash your hands and gently bathe their eyes with damp cotton wool balls to remove any crustiness.
- **Call your doctor**: If you have any concerns about your child's health, or if their condition is getting worse, contact your doctor immediately.

Meningitis

Meningitis is inflammation of the lining around the brain and spinal cord. It can be caused by either viruses or bacteria. Viral meningitis is more common and less serious than bacterial meningitis. Bacterial meningitis can lead to life-threatening blood poisoning, or septicaemia, and should always be treated as a medical emergency.

Did You Know?

Bacterial meningitis is most common in two age groups: children and babies under three, and young people aged between 15 and 24.

Symptoms of meningitis include:

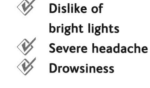

- ☑ Fever
- ☑ Vomiting
- ☑ Stiff neck
- ☑ Confusion
- ☑ Dislike of bright lights
- ☑ Severe headache
- ☑ Drowsiness

In addition you may notice these symptoms of septicaemia:

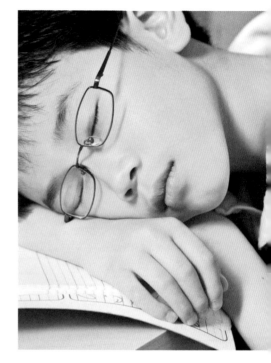

- ☑ Limb, joint or muscle pain
- ☑ Cold hands and feet
- ☑ Pale or mottled skin
- ☑ Breathlessness
- ☑ Rash that does not disappear when you press a glass against it
- ☑ The child appears floppy

Prevention and Treatment

Fortunately, meningitis is extremely rare when compared to other childhood conditions. The best way to prevent meningitis is to make sure that your child's vaccinations are up to date. Routine childhood vaccinations protect against three of the bacteria that can cause meningitis. If a parent has a gut feeling that something is not right they are often correct – do not feel guilty about seeking further medical attention. If you suspect that your child has meningitis, call 999 for an ambulance. At the hospital they may be given:

- ☑ **Antibiotics**: These will kill off any bacteria if the meningitis is bacterial.
- ☑ **Intravenous fluids**: To support your child's body while they recover.
- ☑ **Steroids**: These can help to reduce any swelling around the brain and spinal cord.

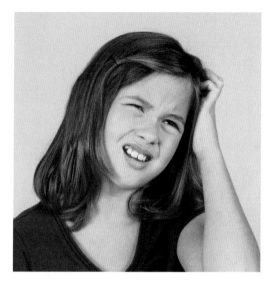

Head Lice

Head lice are tiny grey-brown insects that live in human hair. They survive by sucking small amounts of blood from the scalp. The tiny white eggs are called nits and are glued to the base of hairs. Anyone can catch head lice but they are most common in young children. Head lice can only be caught from head-to-head contact. The main symptom is an itchy scalp. However, children may not notice any symptoms so it's best to check their hair from time to time by wet combing (*see* below).

Prevention and Treatment

Wet comb your child's hair from time to time to see if there are any head lice present and tie long hair back. If you do discover lice, you'll need to act promptly and be persistent, as they are notoriously difficult to get rid of.

- **Wet combing:** Apply a generous amount of conditioner to your child's wet hair at bath time. This means the lice can't hold onto the hairs and you can easily comb them out with a nit comb. Repeat every three days for at least two weeks. Head lice are very contagious, so check the heads of other family members, too.

- **Medicated lotions and shampoos:** These are available from pharmacists, but some head lice are becoming increasingly resistant to them. Follow the instructions on the packet then use a nit comb to comb out the dead lice.

Top Tip

Although there's no scientific evidence to support it, some parents swear by tea tree oil treatments as an effective way to get rid of head lice.

Sore Throat

Sore throats are common in children because they haven't yet built up immunity to all the bacteria and viruses that cause them. Sore throats often, but not always, accompany other infections, such as colds and coughs. Although unpleasant, sore throats are not usually serious and clear up on their own within three to seven days. Symptoms include:

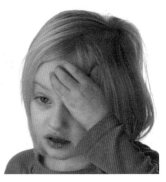

- 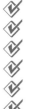 **Soreness and redness at the back of the throat**
- **Enlarged tonsils**
- **Swollen glands in the neck**
- **Pain when swallowing**
- **Fever**
- **Headache**

Prevention and Treatment

Unfortunately sore throats can't be prevented. However, making sure your child eats a healthy diet, exercises regularly and gets plenty of sleep will help them to fight off sore throats and other infections. If they do develop a sore throat, try the following:

- **Children's painkillers:** The correct dose of paracetamol or ibuprofen will help with any pain as well as bringing down fever.
- **Offer cool, soothing foods:** Jelly, yoghurts, soft fruits and ice cream straight from the fridge may help to ease discomfort.
- **Salt-water gargle:** Add a little salt to some lukewarm water. This has healing properties and may help to fight infection. It may be tricky convincing your child of the benefits however...
- **Tonsillectomy:** An operation to remove your child's tonsils will only be considered if they repeatedly get sore throats.

Did You Know?

Doctors rarely prescribe antibiotics for sore throats as research shows that they are no more effective at fighting the symptoms than paracetamol.

Threadworms

Threadworms are small, white thread-like worms that can infest the gut. They are roughly a centimetre (less than half an inch) long and females lay their eggs around the anus at night, causing intense itching. The infected person may then scratch the area causing eggs to stick under their fingernails. These can then be transferred to the mouth and cause re-infestation.

Symptoms

Threadworms cause intense itching around the anus, particularly in the evening and at night, and thus disturbed sleep. In girls the worms may lay their eggs around the vagina and urethra, which may cause symptoms like bedwetting (*see* page 203) or vaginal discharge.

Prevention

Cleanliness is important in order to prevent threadworms. Always wash hands thoroughly with soap and warm water after going to the toilet, change family towels and bedding regularly and vacuum carpets, as threadworm eggs can survive in the environment for up to three weeks.

Treatment

Threadworms are very infectious so everyone in the family should be treated even if they don't have symptoms.

Top Tip

Give children who have threadworms a bath every morning for a few days. This will help to get rid of any eggs that have been laid overnight.

- **Over-the-counter treatments**: All chemists sell palatable tablets that will kill the worms (these are not suitable for babies under three months or pregnant women). The treatment may need to be repeated after two weeks to kill any newly hatched worms.
- **Get rid of the eggs**: Wash bedding, towels, nightclothes and soft toys. Make sure children wear snug-fitting pants in bed.
- **Encourage handwashing**: Make sure everyone washes their hands thoroughly each time they go to the toilet, and keep nails short.

Tooth Decay

Sadly, tooth decay is all too common in children. It happens when poor dental hygiene leads to a build-up of a sticky film called plaque on the teeth. Sugars in food and drink then react with bacteria present in plaque producing acids. It's these acids that eat away at the protective enamel on teeth and eventually cause holes (cavities). Symptoms include:

- **Sensitivity when eating or drinking something hot, cold or sweet**
- **Discoloured spots on the teeth**
- **Bad breath**
- **An unpleasant taste in the mouth**
- **Toothache**

Prevention

Prevention is the key to good dental health:

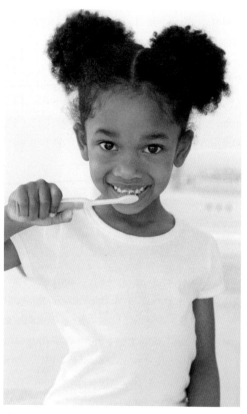

- **Make sure your child brushes with a fluoride toothpaste twice a day**
- **Keep sugary foods and drinks to a minimum**
- **Replace toothbrushes every three months**
- **Make regular visits to the dentist**
- **Limit snacks between meals**
- **Encourage older children to use floss or dental tape every day**
- **Your dentist can apply a protective plastic coating, or sealant, to your child's back teeth if there is no decay yet (you may not find this is available on the NHS in the UK, however)**

Treatment

- **Fillings**: If the decay is not too bad, your dentist can restore the tooth by filling the cavity.
- **Extractions**: If the decay is advanced, your dentist may need to remove the tooth completely.

Ear Infections

Ear infections can be very painful and distressing for children. They usually happen when the middle ear fills with mucus, perhaps during a cold. This mucus can then become infected with bacteria causing pain and inflammation. Repeated ear infections can eventually lead to a chronic condition called glue ear. This may need an operation to clear it up. Symptoms include:

- **Intense pain in the ear**
- **Fever**
- **Slight deafness**
- **In severe cases, the eardrum may rupture and pus, possibly blood-stained, run out of the ear – never clean the ear with a cotton bud; just wipe the pus with a damp flannel on the outside of the ear**

Prevention

- **Chewing gum**: Some Finnish research shows that chewing gum containing xylitol may reduce the risk of children developing ear infections – the act of chewing and swallowing can help clear the middle ear, and xylitol possesses antibacterial properties.
- **Breastfeed**: Children who were bottle-fed are more prone to glue ear.
- **Don't smoke near your child**: Again, this increases the risk of glue ear.

Treatment

Most ear infections clear up within three days without any treatment. Perforated ear drums also usually heal by themselves. However, your child may benefit from:

Plenty of fluids: Offer your child lots of drinks to keep them well hydrated.

 Children's paracetamol or ibuprofen: These will help bring any fever down.

 Nose drops: Your doctor may prescribe drops containing decongestants or antihistamines to reduce swelling in the nose and back of the throat.

 Antibiotics: If the infection is very severe your doctor may prescribe antibiotics, although there is no evidence that they actually help.

Croup

Croup is a common infection that affects the voice box (larynx) and the airways leading to the lungs. It's usually caused by a virus, and is most common in under threes. Croup causes a distinctive seal-like sound when your child coughs. This can be quite alarming, but croup isn't usually serious. It's most likely to occur during the winter months. Symptoms include:

 Seal-like cough

Runny nose

Fever

Croaky voice

Prevention and Treatment

It's hard to prevent the transmission of croup viruses, however it may help to teach your child good personal hygiene – regular hand-washing and so on – and to steer clear of crowded places. If they do get croup, most children can be treated at home:

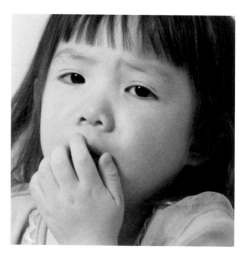

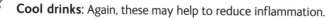 **Cool air**: If it's cool outside, wrap your child up and take them for a stroll. The cool air may help to reduce inflammation in their airway.

Cool drinks: Again, these may help to reduce inflammation.

Did You Know?

Despite researchers' claims that steam inhalation may not work, and the risk of scalds, many doctors still vouch for the benefits of inhaling damp air – for example sitting with the infant in a bathroom fugged-up by running the shower.

- **Anti-fever medication**: If they have a fever, you may want to give them a dose of children's paracetamol or ibuprofen to make them more comfortable.
- **Stay calm**: Croup can be quite distressing for both you and your child. Staying calm will help them to stay relaxed, too.
- **Steroids**: If your child is having difficulty breathing, seek medical help. A doctor can prescribe a steroid medication to reduce inflammation in their airways.

Bedwetting

Occasional bedwetting is perfectly normal up to the age of five, as it takes a while for the nerves supplying the bladder to mature. There are two types of bedwetting in older children. Primary bedwetting is involuntary bedwetting during sleep in a child aged five or over. Secondary bedwetting is when a child wets the bed after a dry period of at least six months. Secondary bedwetting is often linked to stressful events, such as bullying at school. About 15 per cent of children over the age of five experience bedwetting at some point. If your child only wets the bed occasionally, it is probably not a cause for concern. If it happens regularly, it may affect their general wellbeing (by affecting their attitude to sleep-overs and scool trips for instance), so you should get advice from your doctor.

Prevention
- Don't give your child drinks during the couple of hours before bedtime
- Encourage your child to go to the loo before bed
- Make sure your child has easy access to the toilet at night

Don't punish your child for wetting the bed – it may just make things worse

Use a reward system to discourage bedwetting, such as a star chart with coloured stars when your child has a dry night

Treatment

If bedwetting is starting to affect your child's sleep and self-esteem, your doctor may recommend:

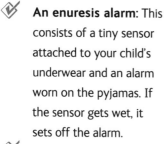 **An enuresis alarm:** This consists of a tiny sensor attached to your child's underwear and an alarm worn on the pyjamas. If the sensor gets wet, it sets off the alarm.

Desmopressin: This drug works by reducing the amount of urine your child produces during the night. It's usually only used in the short term, for example, if you are going away on holiday.

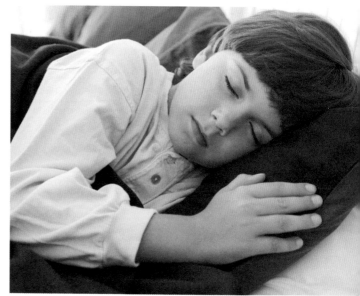

Urinary Tract Infections

Urinary tract infections (UTIs) are fairly common in children. Around 11 per cent of girls and four per cent of boys will have one before they are 16. UTIs can be difficult to diagnose because the symptoms aren't very specific. Sometimes the only symptom may be an unexplained fever. UTIs need to be identified and treated as, left untreated, they can lead to kidney damage. Symptoms include:

- ☑ Unexplained fever
- ☑ Vomiting
- ☑ Needing to wee frequently
- ☑ Tummy pain
- ☑ Pains in the back

Prevention

- ☑ Encourage your child to go to the toilet regularly
- ☑ Encourage them to drink plenty of fluids – this will help flush out any bacteria
- ☑ Avoid synthetic underwear
- ☑ Encourage girls to wipe their bottom from front to back as this will minimize the chance of bacteria entering the urethra
- ☑ Encourage boys to regularly clean their penis – including under their foreskin, where bacteria can build up and then enter the urethra (but only if the foreskin has become retractile, which happens in many boys by two years old but can take longer)

Treatment

If a urine test reveals that your child has an infection, your doctor may recommend the following:

- ☑ **Antibiotics**: UTIs are caused by bacteria, and the antibiotics will kill these off.
- ☑ **Ultrasound**: If the infection doesn't clear up, or if your child has repeated infections, your doctor may refer them for an ultrasound scan to check that everything is in normal working order.

Top Tip

Cranberry juice can help to prevent UTIs by preventing certain types of potentially harmful bacteria from sticking to the walls of the urinary system, so that they can be flushed out of the body more easily.

Slapped Cheek Syndrome

Slapped cheek syndrome is a mild childhood disease that gets its name from the distinctive red rash it sometimes causes on the cheeks. It's caused by the parvovirus and symptoms can be so mild that you may not even know your child has had it. About 60 per cent of adults have had the disease, but many won't be aware that they have been infected. The rash can take up to three weeks to go away. Sometimes there are no symptoms, but in addition to the characteristic red rash on the cheeks (which may spread to the palms of the hands and soles of the feet) your child may have:

 Mild fever    **Sore throat**

Headache   **Stuffy nose**

Prevention and Treatment

As with all infections, the trick is to prevent the virus from spreading, so make sure all family members wash their hands regularly, and avoid places where you know there are infected children. To treat the condition you can offer children's paracetamol or ibuprofen – both can help to ease any fever or aches and pains. Also, it is best to keep your child at home – the main reason being to protect pregnant women, as slapped cheek can cause serious problems for unborn babies.

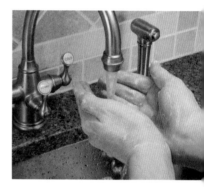

Did You Know?

Children under 16 should not be given aspirin as it can increase the risk of Reye's syndrome, a serious condition that affects the brain and liver.

Asthma

When a person with asthma comes into contact with a substance that irritates their airways, the airways tighten and the lining starts to swell. This makes it difficult to breathe. About one in eleven children have asthma, but about 75 per cent grow out of it. There are effective drugs for asthma and most children achieve a good degree of control over their symptoms. Symptoms include:

- **Coughing (particularly at night)**
- **Phlegm**
- **Wheezing**
- **Shortness of breath**

Prevention

Unfortunately there is no way to stop your child developing asthma. However, you can help to reduce the number of attacks they have:

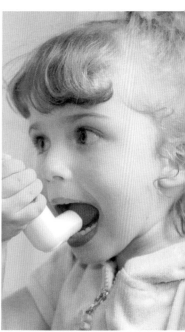

- **Don't smoke near them**
- **Make sure they exercise and eat healthily, to maintain a healthy weight**
- **Avoid possible asthma triggers, such as house dust mites, pollen and animal dander (dead skin scales)**
- **Use an efficient vacuum cleaner and change the filter regularly**
- **Try to avoid fitted carpets if at all possible and ventilate the house regularly**
- **Keep pets out of bedrooms day and night**

Treatment

There is no cure for asthma, but there are effective treatments to control it:

- **Inhalers:** There are two main types of asthma inhalers: relievers and preventers. Your child can take a reliever inhaler whenever they have an attack. Their doctor may also recommend that they take a preventer inhaler every day to keep their symptoms under control.
- **Tablets:** If your child's asthma is severe, they may need to take oral medication as well as their inhalers.

Adenoids

Adenoids are small lumps of tissue at the back of the throat, just above the tonsils. They help to protect the body from bacteria and viruses. Only children have adenoids – by adulthood they have usually disappeared. In some children the adenoids become enlarged, causing pain and interfering with their breathing. If this happens to your child, your doctor may recommend that they have a minor operation to remove them. Symptoms include:

- Pain at the back of the throat
- Noisy breathing and bad breath
- Nasal-sounding speech
- Disturbed sleep
- Glue ear (see page 201)
- Loss of hearing

Prevention and Treatment

Swollen adenoids cannot be prevented. Sometimes children are born with them or they swell up during an infection and then stay enlarged, and allergies can also lead to enlarged adenoids. The minor operation to remove them (an adenoidectomy) only takes about 15 to 30 minutes. Your child will be given a general anaesthetic, but will usually be allowed home the same day. Sometimes the tonsils are removed at the same time as the adenoids. Your child will have a sore throat afterwards, so will need to eat soft or liquid foods for a few days. They will also need to stay off school or nursery for about a week. Your child will not be more prone to infections once the adenoids have been removed.

Attention Deficit and Hyperactivity Disorder (ADHD)

Attention deficit and hyperactivity disorder (ADHD) is the most common behavioural disorder in children. It is thought to affect three to nine per cent of school-age children and can continue into adulthood. It tends to run in families and symptoms usually start to become apparent around age five.

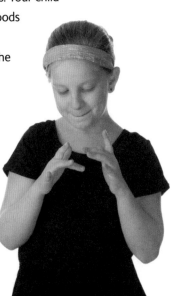

Symptoms vary widely from child to child, but children with ADHD may:

- Be dreamy and inattentive
- Constantly fidget
- Be unable to concentrate on tasks
- Be highly impulsive
- Have no sense of danger

Prevention and Treatment

ADHD cannot be prevented. Treatments for ADHD aim to help children to concentrate better, be less impulsive and feel calmer, and should be a combination of medication and therapy, with schools playing an equally important role:

- **Methylphenidate:** This is the most commonly prescribed medication for ADHD. Your child will normally be given a small dose at first, which can be increased if necessary.
- **Dexamphetamine:** This works in a similar way to methylphenidate. It can be very effective for controlling hyperactivity.
- **Atomoxetine:** Thought to aid concentration and help children control impulses.
- **Behavioural therapy:** This is usually based on a system of rewards and punishments to encourage your child to gain control of their behaviour.

> ## Did You Know?
> Some parents find food supplements, such as omega 3, ginkgo and zinc, helpful for ADHD. Do talk to your doctor before trying them, though.

Autism

People with autism have difficulties communicating with and relating to other people. It's not known what causes autism, but genetics may play a part. There is no 'cure' for autism, but there are plenty of things that can be done to help children with autism thrive. About one in

100 people is thought to be autistic, and it affects four times as many boys as girls. Characteristics include:

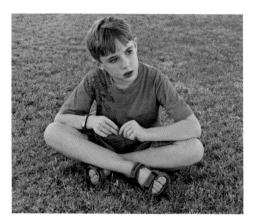

- 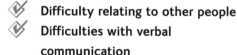 **Difficulty relating to other people**
- **Difficulties with verbal communication**
- **Problems understanding gestures, facial expressions and tones of voice**
- **Fondness of routine**
- **Repetitive behaviours**
- **Over- or undersensitivity to light and noise**

Treatment

There are lots of different forms of help available to children diagnosed with autism:

- **Education:** Some children receive extra support while attending a mainstream school, while others benefit from attending a specialist school for children with autism.
- **Support with socializing:** This may take the form of organized social groups, support with speech and language or behavioural therapy.
- **Medication:** Autism can't be treated medically, but drugs are sometimes used to treat associated behaviours, such as obsessiveness or hyperactivity.
- **Diet:** Some parents find that using food supplements or making changes to their child's diet can have a therapeutic effect. Do check with your doctor before trying this approach.

Dyslexia

Dyslexia is a learning difficulty that affects your child's ability to read, write and spell. It may also influence their short-term memory, maths ability, concentration and organizational skills.

No one knows what causes dyslexia, but it tends to run in families, which suggests a genetic factor. Each child with dyslexia has a unique set of strengths and weaknesses. These may include:

- Difficulty with reading, writing and spelling
- Gets letters and figures the wrong way round
- Difficulty with sequences, such as the days of the week
- Poor concentration
- Poor organization
- Problems with dressing
- Poor sense of direction

- Good verbal and social skills
- Ability to think 'laterally'

Did You Know?

People with dyslexia are often skilled at solving highly complex problems, but may not always be aware of how they did it.

Prevention and Treatment

No one is sure what causes dyslexia, and there is no way to prevent it. If you are concerned about your child, your school or local educational authority can arrange a screening test. If your child is identified as having dyslexia they will need specialist teaching. This will give them the chance to learn in a way that suits them better and at their own pace. Most children will only need a few hours of specialist teaching per week.

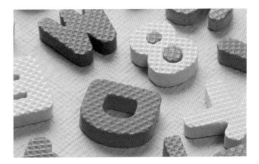

Dyspraxia

In children with dyspraxia, messages from the brain are not passed around the body properly. This means they have problems with movement and coordination, and may also struggle with language and learning. Dyspraxia affects more boys than girls, and up to one in 20 children is thought to have the condition. Characteristics include:

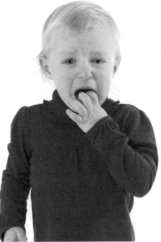

- Difficulty coordinating large-muscle movements like running and jumping
- Problems with small-muscle activities, such as writing, eating and tying up shoelaces
- Poor concentration
- Difficulty picking up new skills
- Difficulty sitting still
- Prone to temper tantrums
- No sense of danger

Prevention and Treatment

No one knows what causes dyspraxia, although it sometimes runs in families. The condition cannot be prevented and there is no treatment for it as such, but there are certain therapies that children with dyspraxia may find helpful:

- **Occupational therapy**: The therapist will help your child manage everyday activities at home and school better.
- **Physiotherapy**: This can help your child learn to control their movements and overcome physical challenges.
- **Speech and language therapy**: If your child struggles with speaking, speech and language therapy may help.
- **Perceptual motor training**: Your child will be set increasingly challenging tasks to stretch their language, visual, motor and hearing skills.

Did You Know?

Having dyspraxia does not affect how intelligent your child is, but it may affect their ability to learn new skills.

The Teen Years

The teen years bring huge changes to a child's life and to that of their parents. First there are the obvious physical changes, and there may be psychological changes, too – adolescents are well known for being moody and self-conscious. Perhaps most challenging are the behavioural changes adolescence brings. This is when many young people start to experiment with new and potentially risky activities, such as smoking, drinking and sex. Whatever challenges are ahead, you'll need to be there for your child and help them to stay as healthy as possible.

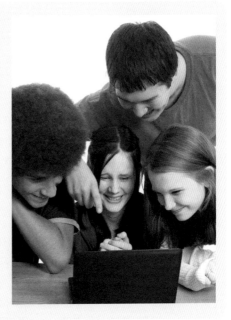

Keeping Your Teenager Healthy

Your teenager probably has more important things on their mind than healthy food and good hygiene. Even so, it's important to encourage them to care for their health during these busy and challenging years.

Nutrition

Teenagers grow fast and tend to be hungry. Stock up on healthy snacks, such as yoghurts, bananas, dried fruit, cheese portions and smoothies, and try to limit crisps, sweets and so on. Encourage your child to have a good breakfast before they go out for the day, and try to involve them in cooking family meals.

Exercise

Older kids are far more likely to exercise regularly if they do something they enjoy. And for girls particularly, it can help if they exercise with friends. Investigate after school clubs, such as yoga or football, and encourage them to join up with other friends. Or check out organized activities, such as sponsored races or gym sessions for young people, in your area. Be a good role model – ordering your child to be more active from the comfort of the sofa simply won't work.

Friendships

Friendships are hugely important to this age group and need to be supported. Encourage your child to invite friends round to the house so that you can meet and get to know them. Make an effort to meet and talk to their parents as well. Don't be tempted to meddle with your child's friendships, but be ready with a listening ear when conflicts come up.

Communication

Adolescent children can be very private, sharing their secrets with friends rather than their parents. You'll need to respect your child's increasing need for privacy, but, at the same time, keep the lines of communication open. The best time for conversations is when you are together, but occupied – when out shopping, for example, or clearing up the kitchen. General conversation openers like, 'How are you doing?' may be more productive than specific questions like, 'What did you do at school today?'

Mood swings

With all those hormones raging around their body and the new challenges that adolescence brings, mood swings are inevitable during your child's teen years. Although it's not always easy, try to keep some perspective and a sense of humour. Mood swings should tail off as your child gets older. Do be prepared to put your foot down when their behaviour is really unacceptable.

Sleep

Teenagers need about nine hours sleep a night. That means, if your child gets up at seven o'clock during the week, they'll need to be asleep by about 10 o'clock. Make sure your teenager heads for bed at a decent hour every weeknight, and also discourage them from staying up too late at the weekend. Research shows that having electronic devices like mobile phones, computers and TVs in their room can interfere with teenagers' sleep, so consider banning these from their bedroom after a certain time.

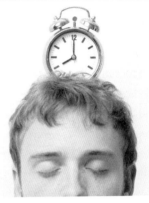

Alcohol

There's no 'right' age for children to start drinking alcohol, but some experts recommend that children under 15 do not drink alcohol at all. Teenagers are more vulnerable to the harmful effects of alcohol than adults, so heavy drinking should definitely be discouraged. One of the best things you can do is demonstrate responsible, moderate drinking to your teen. If they do have a binge, try to be matter of fact and explain the possible risks. Explain how you feel and encourage them to talk about why it happened.

Drugs

Make sure you are informed about drugs so that you can talk confidently about them with your child if the need arises. It's natural to feel anxious if you think your child is taking drugs, but it's important not to panic and go on the offensive. Talk to your child and help them think through the possible consequences. Let them know you are there to help them if they get into difficulties. Remember – there's no evidence that teenagers who experiment with drugs go on to become regular users.

Sex and Relationships

Believe it or not, research shows that teenagers do actually want to talk to their mums and dads about sex and relationships. It doesn't have to be one big 'birds and bees' talk. It's more a case of exploiting opportunities that come up naturally. Watching a TV programme that raises sexual or relationship issues, for example, may give you a natural opener. Ask your child what they think. Or, if their friends are starting to have relationships, ask how they feel about that. Let them know that you are there to answer questions and help them deal with any problems that arise.

School

School can be a source of stress to teenagers as well as a source of friendship and learning. Let your child know that you are there for them if they ever need to talk about problems at school. Make links with other parents so that you have an overview of what's going on for your child and their friends. Building a relationship with the school, perhaps by joining the Parent Teachers Association, is another good way to be in the know and support your child.

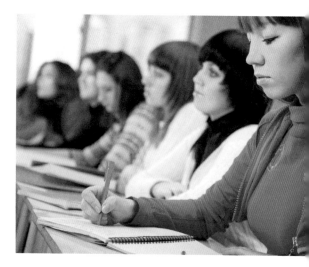

Teenage Health Problems

Hormonal changes in your teenager's body can bring upsetting new health problems, such as acne and body odour. Teenagers are also more prone to certain conditions, such as hay fever or glandular fever, than young children so it's important to be on the lookout for them, too.

Acne

Acne – spots that appear on the face, back and chest – isn't a serious condition, but can have a serious effect on a self-conscious teenager's self-esteem. In girls it's usually worst between the ages of 14 and 17. In boys the condition is most common between 16 and 19. Luckily, there are effective treatments available on prescription from your doctor. Despite what you or your child may hear, changing their diet, sunbathing and squeezing spots won't help to improve the condition.

Period pain

Painful periods are particularly common in teenage girls and young women. It's not known why. The pain is caused by chemicals called prostaglandins, which make the womb contract and expel its lining each month. Warmth can help to ease the pain, so encourage your daughter to have a warm bath or cuddle up with a hot water bottle. A gentle massage may help, as will wearing loose clothing. Some young women find gentle exercise, such as yoga, walking or swimming, useful. Regular painkillers like paracetamol or ibuprofen may help, too. If the pain is particularly severe, it can be treated with the contraceptive pill – speak to your doctor.

Body odour

Body odour is a common teenage problem, as many parents of teenagers will confirm. Smelly armpits and feet are caused by sweat being broken down by bacteria into acids. It's these acids that produce the odour. Teenage boys are more likely to suffer from body odour than girls simply because they produce more sweat. Washing daily and using a deodorant on clean armpits should be enough to control the problem. Washing feet thoroughly with soap and water and changing socks daily should stop feet getting smelly. Cotton or wool socks are best, and avoid shoes made of synthetic materials.

Top Tip

Another way to get rid of the bacteria that cause smelly feet is to wipe them all over with a cotton wool ball soaked in surgical spirit. Surgical spirit is available from your local chemist.

Hay fever

Hay fever is an allergy to pollen in the air. Symptoms usually start in the early teens and peak during the twenties. For many teenagers one of the worst things about hay fever is that it tends to coincide with the exam period. Your child may have to cope with sneezing, itchy eyes and a stuffy nose at the same time as their GCSEs or A levels. The first-line treatment of hay fever is usually antihistamine tablets or nasal sprays. These will help with itching and sneezing by reducing the amount of itch-inducing histamine. Antihistamine eye drops can relieve itchy and swollen eyes. If necessary, your doctor can also prescribe a steroid nasal spray or eye drops. These are most effective if you start using them a couple of weeks before symptoms usually begin and use them regularly throughout the hay-fever season.

Glandular Fever

Glandular fever can affect people of any age, but is most common in teenagers. It's caused by the Epstein-Barr virus, which is spread by saliva. That's why glandular fever is sometimes known as kissing disease. Symptoms include sore throat, fever, swollen glands in the neck or armpits, fatigue and weakness. Most of the symptoms will clear up after four to six weeks, but feelings of fatigue can last for up to six months. There is no cure for glandular fever, but it's important that your child gets plenty of rest as this will speed up their recovery. Gargling with salt water may help a sore throat, while paracetamol or ibuprofen can help to control fever. Make sure your child has plenty of fluids, too.

Did You Know?

Even though the Epstein-Barr virus is contagious, there's no need to keep your child away from other people while they're ill as 90 per cent of people will already have had the virus.

Eating Disorders

Eating disorders happen when people start to control their food intake as a way to relieve stress or cope with painful situations or feelings. Anyone can develop an eating disorder, but young women between the ages of 15 and 25 are most vulnerable. There are several kinds of eating disorder, but anorexia and bulimia are the most common. Signs include pronounced weight loss, intolerance of cold, loss of periods, compulsive behaviour, exhaustion, and dry skin and hair. Helping a child with an eating disorder can be extremely distressing and difficult as they often deny there is a problem and resist treatment. Getting fully informed about the nature of eating disorders and seeking out specialist medical help early are good places to start.

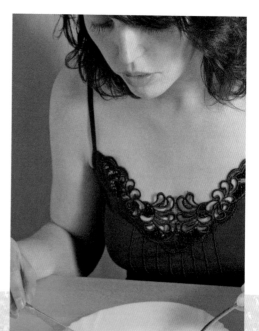

Checklist

- ☑ **Vaccinations**: Make sure your baby has all their routine vaccinations to protect them against potentially serious diseases like meningitis and measles.
- ☑ **Protect your child from smoke**: Never smoke during pregnancy or near your child.
- ☑ **Breastfeeding benefits**: Breastfeeding your baby exclusively for six months can help to prevent allergies, such as peanut allergy, and infections, such as gastroenteritis.
- ☑ **Hygiene**: Regular handwashing by all members of the family, especially after going to the loo, is one of the best ways to prevent the spread of infections.
- ☑ **Vulnerability**: Minor infections, such as colds and tummy upsets, are very common in babies and young children. That's because their immune systems aren't fully developed yet.
- ☑ **Always trust your instincts**: As parents, you know your child far better than anyone else and it's important to seek medical help if you are at all concerned about their health or wellbeing.
- ☑ **Fighting fit**: Plenty of sleep, regular exercise and a well-balanced diet are the best ways to keep your child's body in top disease-fighting condition.
- ☑ **Teen troubles**: During the teenage years, be prepared to support your child through a new set of health problems, such as acne, period pain and hay fever.

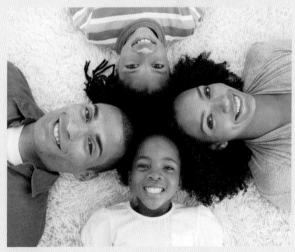

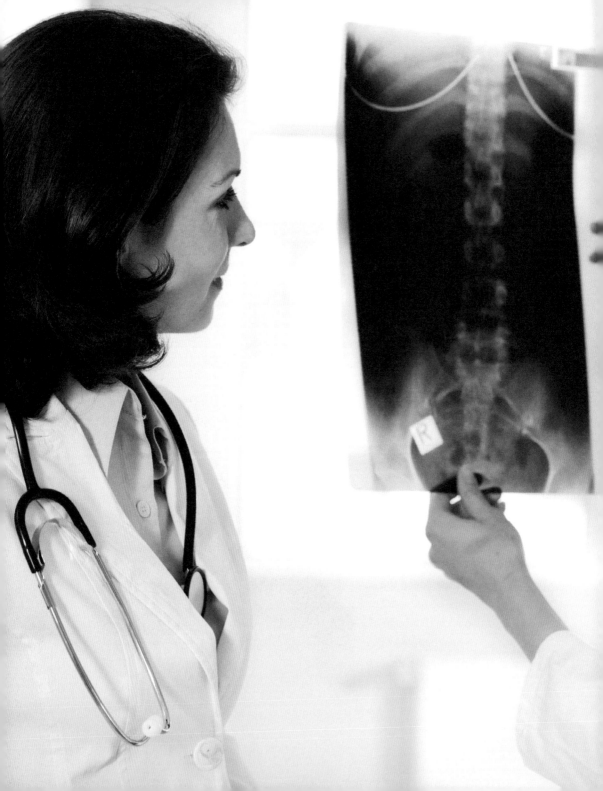

Emergencies
& First Aid

Life-threatening Situations

Thousands of people die every year as a result of medical emergencies such as heart attack, stroke, falls or car accidents. Doctors believe many could survive if first aid was given before the emergency services arrive. There is a relatively short time period – often called the 'Golden Hour' – after an emergency occurs when the patient has most to gain from interventions. Learning the techniques in this section could help you save a life. However, this advice does not replace formal first-aid training. *See also* page 142 for what to do if someone has a hypoglycaemic attack.

If Someone Has Collapsed

If you come across someone who has collapsed – perhaps after an accident or heart attack; first of all make sure the patient is safe and find out whether they are conscious. Shout 'Can you hear me? Can you open your eyes?' and shake them by the shoulder. Have concern for your own safety too – check that the patient is not in contact with any live electrical risk, and be aware of fire risk and transport dangers.

If the Patient Responds

If you get a response, call the emergency services (999, or 911 if you are in the US, for example) for an ambulance immediately, if needed. While you are waiting, treat any obvious medical condition (such as bleeding) and monitor their pulse (you can do this by placing two fingers on one side of their voice box), breathing and level of responsiveness until help arrives.

Top Tip

Check your own pulse at the same time as the patient's, to avoid mistaking your own pulse for theirs.

No Response: ABC

If the patient doesn't respond, call for 999

backup and leave the patient in the position found, taking care to ensure their airway (mouth) is clear (to do this see A for Airways below). Follow the ABC (Airways, Breathing, Circulation) procedures below. The ABC checklist is an easy way to remember what to do if a patient is unconscious and not responding.

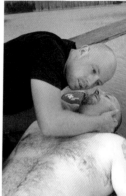

 A = Open the Airways: It's crucial to ensure the patient's airways are open to stop them swallowing their tongue or choking on vomit or fluids. To do this put one hand on the patient's forehead and gently tilt the head back, then lift the chin using two fingers.

 B = Check Breathing: Spend no more than 10 seconds assessing whether the patient is breathing by checking to see if their chest is rising and falling, feeling for their breath against your cheek and listening out for the signs of normal breathing. If they are breathing normally they should be placed in the recovery position (*see* below) and any other life-threatening condition (such as bleeding) should be treated.

 C = Aid Circulation: Performing cardiopulmonary resuscitation (CPR – *see* page 226) is only necessary if the patient isn't breathing – and you should call 999 immediately if you find this to be the case. The purpose of CPR is to breathe for the patient and manually send oxygen around the body by pressing on the chest and performing mouth-to-mouth resuscitation. This can prevent brain damage caused by oxygen starvation.

The Recovery Position

This is the name for the ideal position for an unconscious casualty who is still breathing but not suffering from any other life-threatening conditions. Here's how:

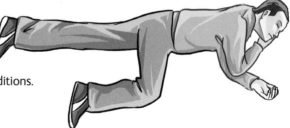

 Move the casualty onto their side
 Their chin should be tilted forward and their hand adjusted under their cheek

☑ You should check the casualty can't roll backwards – pulling their top knee forwards helps this

☑ Keep checking they are breathing and feel their pulse (*see* page 224) continuously

☑ If their injuries allow, the casualty should be turned onto their other side in 30 minutes

The Recovery Position in Babies Under One

A baby who is unconscious but still breathing, with no other life-threatening injuries, should be cradled in your arms with their head tilted downwards to prevent choking on the tongue or breathing in vomit. Monitor and record their pulse, breathing and how responsive they are until the emergency services arrive.

CPR

There is a set procedure for CPR, used when the patient is not breathing:

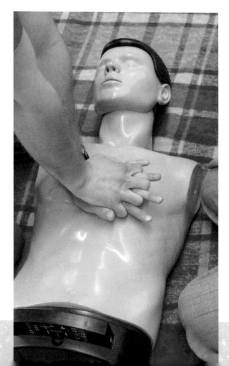

☑ **Place hands**: Put the heel of your hand in the middle of the chest, place your other hand on top and interlock fingers.

☑ **Check position**: Your arms should be straight and your fingers raised off the chest.

☑ **Press and release**: Press down vertically 4–5 cm (1½–2 inches) and then release the pressure, keeping your hands in place. This squeezes blood out of the heart and into body tissues.

☑ **Repeat**: Repeat this movement 30 times at a rate of 100 per minute.

☑ **Give breath**: Then give two breaths. To do this you need to keep the airway open and pinch the nose closed. Take a deep breath and blow into the patient's mouth until you see their chest rising. Remove your mouth, let the chest fall and repeat again.

 If the patient still isn't breathing: Perform more chest compressions – up to 30 – and repeat more mouth to mouth rescue breaths.

 Continue: Keep doing this until either the patient starts breathing normally or emergency services arrive to take over.

Top Tip

Don't give up. Patients rarely respond to CPR (Cardio Pulmonary Resuscitation) straight away so persevere.

What To Do If a Baby Stops Breathing

In this situation you should call emergency services immediately if you have someone with you, or:

 Give the kiss of life: If you are alone, give five rescue breaths first then ring the emergency services. Make sure their mouth is open, seal your lips around the baby's mouth and nose and blow air gently into the lungs, checking the chest is rising as you breathe. As the chest rises, stop your breaths and allow it to fall and repeat five times.

Give 30 chest compressions: Pressing down with your fingers to approximately one third of the depth of their chest (*see* CPR, page 226). After the compressions give two rescue breaths and begin compressions again. Do not stop until help arrives.

Treating Shock

If you arrive at the scene of a serious road accident or other emergency, you are likely to find casualties suffering from shock. Patients who have suffered a heart attack may also display shock symptoms, because their heart has been damaged and is not working properly. Shock is the body's physical response to trauma.

Symptoms

- A fast, weak pulse
- Shallow fast breathing
- Grey or pale pallor
- Clammy, cold, sweaty skin
- Severe thirst
- Dizziness and/or weakness
- Feeling sick and/or vomiting

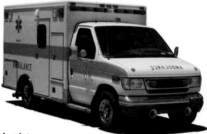

Treatment

- Call an ambulance and reassure the patient
- Treat any obvious injuries
- Lay them on a blanket to keep them warm
- Make them comfortable by loosening any tight clothing
- Raise and support their legs above the level of their heart
- DON'T give anything to eat or drink in case they need an anaesthetic for an operation later on

Dealing With Heavy Blood Loss

If someone is bleeding heavily your first aim must be to stop the blood flow. Call 999.

Is There an Object Embedded in the Wound?

Large objects, like a knife or piece of glass, should not be pulled out of the wound. Smaller objects can be washed out with water.

Apply Pressure

Apply direct pressure to the wound (if no object is embedded) with your fingers (wearing sterile gloves if possible to prevent risk of infection), a pad or with a clean cloth, until emergency services arrive. Raise and support any injured limb.

Treat Shock

Treat the casualty for shock (see 227).

Bandage the Dressing

Keep the dressing or pad in place with firm bandaging to stem the bleeding. If blood seeps through, add another layer on top – but do not remove what you have already applied.

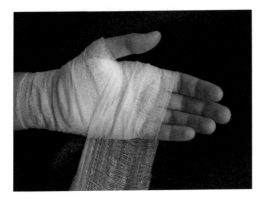

Did You Know?

If shock is not treated promptly the patient can become restless and aggressive, appear to gasp for breath and lose consciousness. The heart may stop. Continue checking vital signs and be prepared to perform CPR if necessary.

Treating a Nosebleed

Nosebleeds can cause rapid blood loss. Treat by:

 Sitting the patient down and putting their head forwards to allow blood to drain from the nostrils

Pinch the end of the nose and ask the patient to breathe through their nose

After 10 minutes release the pressure to check if bleeding has stopped

If bleeding hasn't stopped reapply pressure for up to two further periods of 10 minutes. If possible, put an ice cube in a plastic bag and place on the side of the nose that is bleeding. If bleeding continues seek emergency medical advice

Important

Thin and watery blood loss can be a sign of fluids leaking from around the brain because of a skull fracture (*see* Head Injuries, page 233).

Treating Burns

Burns and scalds are caused by skin coming into contact with fire, electricity, hot liquids or chemicals. Burns can cause rapid fluid loss. In severe cases permanent nerve damage may occur and layers of tissue die, so a skin graft is required.

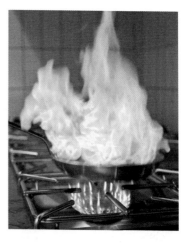

Step-by-step Treatment

- **Remove the patient's clothing**: Do this carefully, unless it is stuck (in which case you may need to wait for more expert help).
- **Cool the skin with cold water**: Put skin under cool (not very cold or icy) running water for a minimum of 10 minutes.
- **Cover with a sterile dressing**: Plastic kitchen film is a good choice for dressing a burn. Avoid cotton wool or fluffy-type dressings and material.
- **Do NOT apply creams, butter or ice**: Ointments and creams will not necessarily be effective and may need to be removed by medical staff to allow them to assess the burn.
- **Seek medical help**: Any burn bigger than a 50p coin needs checking. A doctor or nurse can assess the depth and extent of skin damage and in the most severe case decide if skin grafts are needed. If the patient has lost lots of fluid they may need to be kept hydrated on a drip or treated at a specialist burns unit.

Chemical Burns

In cases of chemical burns remove contaminated clothing and brush the chemical off the skin if it is powder form, then rinse the skin with water for a minimum of 20 minutes, taking care not to come into contact with the chemicals yourself.

Choking

When the throat becomes obstructed with an object (usually food) it can be life-threatening as the patient's airways become blocked and they are unable to breathe. It is common in babies and young children, so one effective preventative measure is to never let children eat and play at the same time. Mild obstructions should be able to be cleared by coughing, but if the person is unable to cough up the object and is struggling to breathe, you need to take urgent action:

What to Do in Severe Cases

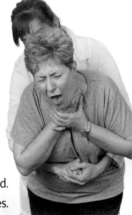

- **Back blows:** Give up to five back blows on the casualty between the shoulder blades, using the heel of your hand. Check the mouth each time to see if the object has become dislodged.
- **Abdominal thrusts:** If the object is still stuck in the throat, you need to give up to five abdominal thrusts (also known as the Heimlich manoeuvre). Stand behind the patient, place your arms round their waist and bend forward. Put your clenched fist above the belly button with your other hand on top and pull it inwards and upwards in a hard upright movement, again checking the mouth after each one to see if the object has become dislodged.
- **Combination:** Continue back blows and abdominal thrusts for three cycles. If the object is still causing choking then call 999 and continue with back blows and thrust and resuscitate if necessary (*see ABC, page 224*).

Choking in a Baby Under One

- **Back blows:** Lay the baby along your forearm with their head down and support their back and head. Give five back blows between the shoulder blades with the heel of your hand – checking between each blow to see if the object has been dislodged.
- **Chest thrusts:** If they are still choking, turn them onto their back and give up to five chest thrusts. Push inwards and upwards with two fingers against the baby's breastbone one finger's breadth below the nipple line. Check after each one to see if the obstruction has been cleared. Call 999 if the object is not dislodged after three cycles and then continue.

Anaphylactic Shock

This is a severe type of allergic reaction caused by an insect sting, eating certain foods or coming into contact with a certain material. Common triggers can include wasp and bee stings, shellfish, peanuts and nuts, eggs, dairy products, sesame, penicillin and aspirin and latex.

Symptoms

The symptoms can be life-threatening and include:

- Breathing difficulties
- Wheezing
- Swelling of the face, neck, hands or feet
- Swelling of the tongue
- Increased pulse
- Stomach pains, vomiting, diarrhoea
- Blotchy red skin and/or an itchy rash (hives)
- Sudden feeling of weakness (caused by drop in blood pressure)
- Unconsciousness and collapse

How to Treat Anaphylactic Shock

Firstly, call 999. Then check to see if they have an EpiPen® – if the patient knows they have an allergy they may be carrying a pre-loaded syringe containing epinephrine (adrenaline), which acts quickly to constrict blood vessels and relax smooth muscles in the lungs to improve breathing, stimulate heartbeat and stop swelling. Help them into a sitting position and wait for help to arrive. If you or one of the family has an EpiPen, ensure that you keep an eye on the expiry date as they tend to have a short lifespan.

Electrocution

Tissues can be damaged by the passage of electricity and the heat this releases as it passes through the body. Electrocution can cause burn injuries to the muscles, nerves and skin as well as cardiac arrhythmia (irregular heart beat) and cardio-respiratory arrest (heart and breathing stop). High voltages of 480 volts and above are the most dangerous.

First Aid for Electrocution

 Turn off the power: Unless the power supply has been turned off, do not touch the victim.

 Avoid moisture: Don't touch the victim with anything wet.

 Disconnect: If you can't pull out the plug, stand on a dry object such as a telephone directory and push the victim away from the electrical source with a broom.

 ABC: Once the victim is disconnected from the source of electricity assess them using the ABC criteria: call 999 and begin CPR if necessary, or if the victim is breathing place them in the recovery position (*see* pages 225–26). Follow first-aid advice for burns and shock (*see* pages 230 and 227).

Drowning

If you pull someone unconscious from the water, lay them down on land and assess them according to the ABC procedures (*see* page 224). If they have stopped breathing and have no pulse perform CPR (*see* page 226).

CPR for Drowning

The only difference is that you need to give *FIVE* rescue breaths initially and perform CPR for one minute before calling 999, and then continue with CPR until help arrives.

Head Injuries: Cerebral Compression

All head injuries are potentially dangerous because of the risk that the brain has been injured or the skull fractured. There is a risk the patient may have sustained a life-threatening cerebral compression, which is one of the most severe types of head injury. Cerebral compression follows a build-up of pressure in the brain caused by bleeding or swelling of brain tissue. Warning signs to look out for include:

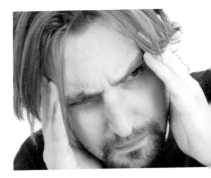

- Unconsciousness
- Patient complaining of a painful headache
- Unequal pupil size
- Weakness or even paralysis down one side
- Laboured breathing
- Slow pulse
- Irritability
- Patient seems confused or disorientated
- High temperature/fever

What You Can Do

First of all ring emergency services backup, as it's likely the patient will need surgery as soon as possible. If the patient is conscious, support them in a comfortable position, check their breathing, pulse and responsiveness. If they are unconscious, make sure their airway is open, monitor their breathing and wait for help.

Head Injuries: Fractured Skull

Skull fractures can be dangerous because it means the brain may be damaged by bleeding or fractured bone. The key warning sign of a fractured skull is *clear fluid leaking from ear or nose*, as this indicates fluid is leaking from the brain. Other symptoms can include:

- Soft area of depression on skull
- Blood in the whites of the eyes

- Bruising around the eyes
- Deterioration in responsiveness

Treatment

This depends on whether the patient is conscious or unconscious.

- **Conscious**: Help them to lie down but be careful not to turn their head because of the likelihood of neck/spinal injury and monitor vital signs until emergency help arrives. Also apply pressure to control bleeding from the scalp.
- **Unconscious**: Dial 999 and keep their airways open (*see* page 225), monitor vital signs and be prepared to give chest compressions if their heart stops.

Head Injuries: Concussion

This is a less serious head injury caused by the brain being shaken within the skull, causing a short period of impaired consciousness lasting usually no more than a few minutes. Dizziness, nausea and short-term memory loss may also occur.

Treatment

Follow the AVPU code below and be sure to monitor vital signs; observe for an extended period and get medical advice if the patient reports blurred vision or headache.

 A: Check whether the patient is alert, has eyes open and can answer questions.

 V: Observe whether the patient responds to voice command.

 P: Do they respond to pain?

 U: Is the patient unresponsive?

Heart Attack

Heart attacks can prove fatal and need urgent attention.
Symptoms can vary but commonly include:

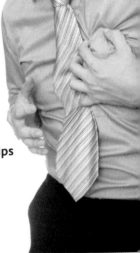

- Severe and crushing pain in the centre of the chest
- Pain travelling to the jaw, neck, arms and wrist
- Clamminess and sweating
- Grey pale skin and blue lips
- Nausea
- Indigestion-like pain
- Breathlessness
- Collapse

Treatment

If you suspect someone is having a heart attack, call 999 and do the following:

 If they are conscious: Sit them in a 75 degree angle, with knees bent and call an ambulance. Give them a 300 mg aspirin tablet to chew - this will help stop the blood clots in the arteries getting any bigger. If they have angina medication, make sure they take it and keep checking pulse, breathing etc. until the ambulance arrives.

If they become unconscious: Keep their airways open using the ABC procedure and be ready to start CPR (*see* pages 225 and 226).

Stroke

A stroke can be a life-threatening event which occurs when the blood supply to the brain is interrupted – they can either be ischaemic, in which a blood clot blocks one of the arteries in your brain, or haemorrhagic, where one of the blood vessels in your brain bursts. You are at increased risk of a stroke if you are elderly, suffer high blood pressure, smoke or are diabetic. Stroke is one of those serious illnesses where prompt emergency care can make all the difference, so call the emergency services if you suspect one.

Symptoms

These can include:

- **One-sided body or facial weakness, numbness or paralysis/droopiness, such as of the eye or mouth**
- **Inability to raise both arms above their head and keep them there**
- **Slurred speech**
- **Blurred vision**
- **Confusion**
- **Severe headache**
- **Dizziness, balance and coordination problems**
- **Swallowing difficulties and loss of consciousness**

Treatment

If you suspect a stroke call the emergency services immediately. It's important NOT to give anyone who is having a stroke any food or water: stroke can often cause problems with the swallow function and as a result there is a risk that food and drink may get into the windpipe and then the lungs. Keep the patient's airways open until help arrives. The main treatment is thrombolytic (clot-busting) drugs which need to be administered by doctors or paramedics within three hours. Other treatments include blood pressure medication, statins and surgery (see page 133).

No Aspirin

You *SHOULD NOT* give aspirin to stroke victims; aspirin lowers the risk of blood clots forming and could help individuals who have a clot, but if they are suffering from a bleed, giving them aspirin could be fatal. The only way to check if a person is having a clot or bleed is by brain scan – so do not give aspirin.

Asthma Attack

Asthma is a condition where breathing becomes difficult because of narrowing of the airways when muscles go into spasm. An asthma attack can be triggered by allergies, cold weather, smoke and exercise. Symptoms can include difficulty in breathing, wheezing, coughing and a grey-blue tinge to earlobes, lips and nail beds because of oxygen deprivation.

Treatment
Initially try the following:

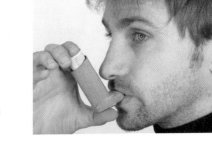

- Keep the patient calm and give reassurance
- If they are asthmatic they should be carrying a blue reliever inhaler, tell them to use it
- Ask them to breathe slowly and deeply if they can
- Ask them to lean forward with arms resting on a table or chair – do not lie down
- If symptoms don't improve after 5 minutes of using a reliever inhaler seek urgent medical attention and repeat use of the inhaler every five to 10 minutes until help arrives

First Aid for Everyday Health Problems

This section is designed to act as a handy reference self-help guide for common health ailments like bites and stings, sprains and bruising, cramps and nosebleeds. Be aware that some comparatively minor injuries or bites and stings can have potentially fatal consequences though.

Bruises

Bruises develop after your body comes into collision with a person or object. This can cause tiny blood vessels under the skin to leak blood, causing swelling, discolouration and pain. Skin tends to turn in sequence from red/purple, to blue/black, to green/yellow and then light-brown over a 14-day period. There is usually some pain, swelling and tenderness initially.

Treatment

✔ **Cold:** Apply an icepack or cold compress such as a bag of peas from the freezer wrapped in a cloth; as soon as possible can reduce swelling and the size of the blood vessels.

✔ **Seek help:** See a doctor if your bruising has not subsided within two weeks as it could mean a haematoma (blood pooling under the skin) has developed which may need treatment.

Top Tip

Natural remedies for bruises include witchhazel and arnica.

Cuts and Grazes

Most cuts and tears in the skin don't need any medical attention, likewise grazes which are caused by the skin being scraped against a hard surface. Most cuts and grazes will heal quickly.

Clean the wound with running water, pat dry with a clean towel. Then apply a plaster and sterile dressing. If needed, take a painkiller.

Cuts: When To Get Medical Help

There are times when you may need medical help for cuts, including:

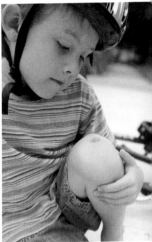

- **If the injury is large and deep – especially deep cuts to the palm of the hand or sole of the foot**
- **If blood is pouring from the wound and it doesn't stop after five minutes (go straight to A and E). (*See also*, Dealing With Heavy Blood Loss, page 228).**
- **The edges of the cut cannot be brought together, such as when pulled apart by movement because it is on a crease or a joint**
- **There is an object embedded in the cut (*do not remove*)**
- **The skin has been broken by a bite**
- **The cut is accompanied by numbness**
- **There is a risk that the cut is infected with bacteria from soil or manure, for example**
- **It can't be covered with a sticking plaster**
- **It is oozing with pus, swollen or painful, indicating infection**

Treatment Options For Severe Cuts And Grazes

If your wound is larger than 5 cm (2 inches) you will need a surgical stitch, done under a local anaesthetic. Smaller wounds are closed with skin glue or steri-strips.

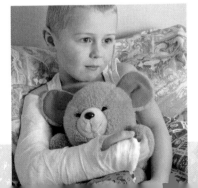

Broken Bones

If you've had a fall or accident, you might have broken a bone, referred to by medics as a fracture. These vary in severity but all need medical attention.

Symptoms

It can be difficult to distinguish a break from a joint or muscle problem. Here are some of the telltale warning signs that you may have broken a bone:

 Bone bent/sticking out
at a funny angle

 Can't bear weight on it

 Grinding sensation

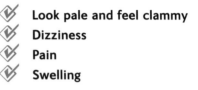 Look pale and feel clammy

Dizziness

Pain

Swelling

If You Suspect a Broken Bone

A fracture will be diagnosed by an X-ray at hospital, but until you get there:

 Keep the patient still: Ideally don't move the casualty (unless it's crucial to get them out of danger) until a splint has been applied.

Make a splint: In an emergency you should bandage a broken leg to the other leg at the knee and ankle to give makeshift support or improvise a sling for a broken arm.

Make them comfy: Try to make the casualty comfortable and call 999.

Treat for any shock symptoms: *See page 227.*

Further Treatment

At the hospital you will usually need an operation to re-align the end of the broken bone. It will then be immobilized either in a plaster cast, or steel rods, or metal plates and screws for two to eight weeks, depending on how severe the break is.

Sprains and Strains

These can be tricky to distinguish from each other, but as a general rule of thumb a sprain involves ligaments (a band of tissue that connects bones to each other in a joint) and a strain is an injury to a muscle or tendon and tends to happen when stretched, twisted or torn, usually by playing sport.

Symptoms

Symptoms for sprains and strains are very similar, except that with sprains the pain tends to be around the joint, while with strains it tends to be in the muscle. Both can have the following symptoms:

 Inability to bear weight   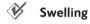 **Swelling**

Bruising and tenderness

Treatment

The best painkillers for sprains and strains are paracetamol or codeine; some organizations recommend avoiding ibuprofen or other anti-inflammatories for the first 48 hours because of theoretical concerns that they may impair healing (some inflammation arguably being necessary for the healing process). And follow the RICE procedure below:

 R: Rest the injured ligament or muscle (for between 48 and 72 hours usually)

I: Ice (wrapped in a towel) should be applied for 15–20 minutes, every 2–3 hours for 48–72 hours

C: Comfortably support the injury with a bandage or soft padding

E: Elevate the injured part

After the initial injury, doctors say you should avoid HARM for 72 hours:

 H: Heat (hot baths etc.)

A: Alcohol

R: Running

M: Massage

Further Treatment

Get medical help if the patient can't bear weight, experiences numbness, cannot move the joint or muscle, or if pain has not got any better after four hours.

Back Injuries

These can be potentially very serious because the spinal cord in the back contains nerves which communicate with the brain about the control of bodily functions. Always suspect a spinal injury if:

 The patient has fallen awkwardly from a height

Has a head injury

Is experiencing loss of feeling or movement

Treatment

Try to keep the patient still (see page 240) and support their head, neck and shoulders with rolled up coats or blankets, before summoning emergency help. Protect the patient from getting cold with further coats or blankets.

Cramp

Muscle cramps are extremely common. One third of the over 60s suffer cramp. They are also common in pregnant women and children over 12. Often there is no obvious cause; but muscle cramps may follow strenuous exercise or be a side effect of medication (such as the cholesterol-lowering drugs statins).

Symptoms

A muscle goes into painful spasm, usually in the calf, thigh muscle or the foot

The muscle that is in spasm feels hard and tender

The experience usually lasts no longer than 10 minutes

It commonly happens when you are in bed resting or sleeping

Treatment

Painkillers don't take effect until after a cramp has stopped so are not much use for leg cramps.

You can relieve your symptoms with stretching exercises, such as straightening your leg and bending the ankle backwards, and walking on tiptoes.

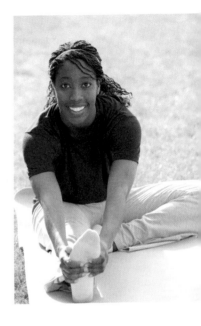

Prevention

Tips for preventing leg cramps include:

- Supporting your toes with a pillow while you sleep
- Taking quinine or sipping tonic water
- Sleeping under loose bed covers and lying with your toes hanging over the edge of the bed
- Keep well hydrated before, during and after exercise
- Warm up and warm down before and after exercise
- Talk to your doctor about changing your medication if you suspect it is to blame

Fainting

Fainting is common and is a major cause of falls amongst the elderly. It is caused by a temporary disruption to the blood supply to the brain. The medical name for this is syncope and it has a number of causes, including irregular heartbeat conditions, which can sometimes

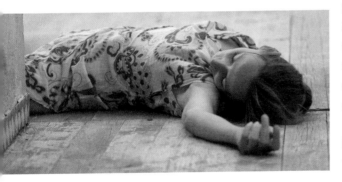

prove fatal if not corrected. For this reason it is recommended that anyone who has a blackout be monitored with a 12-lead electrocardiogram (ECG) to check for an abnormal heart rhythm.

Symptoms

These can include temporary loss of

consciousness and falling to the floor. The person may also turn deathly pale and you may notice limb twitching and incontinence.

First Aid Treatment

The patient should wake fairly quickly and may remember blacking out and appear to recover quickly. You can help them by:

- ☑ Laying them down flat and loosening their clothing
- ☑ Checking their airways are clear and that they are still breathing and have a pulse (*see* page 224)
- ☑ Moving them to the recovery position (*see* page 225) to avoid the risk of them inhaling vomit or choking on their tongue
- ☑ Calling 999 if they don't recover consciousness

Fits and Seizures

Epileptic seizures are caused by recurrent disturbances in electrical activity in the brain (*see* Epilepsy, page 58). Usually, the patient suddenly loses consciousness or blacks out temporarily. Other symptoms include:

- ☑ Arching or rigid back
- ☑ Violent involuntary limb twitching
- ☑ Frothing of saliva of the mouth
- ☑ Jaw clenching or tongue biting (which may cause bleeding from the mouth)
- ☑ Loss of bladder and bowel control
- ☑ Noisy breathing

Top Tip

When to dial 999: Most seizures will be over quickly and typically don't last longer than five minutes (if they do you should call 999 immediately).

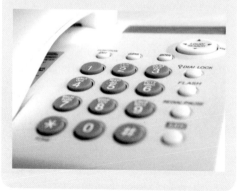

First Aid Treatment

 Safety: Aim to make the patient safe by clearing a space around them so they don't injure themselves when their limbs are flailing.

Protect the head: If you can, place soft padding – such as a towel, coat or blanket – around the patient's head.

Check airways: When the seizure has finished, check the patient's airway is clear and that they're breathing and have a pulse. If they don't have any vital signs – perform CPR (*see* page 226) and call 999.

If they're conscious: Move them into the recovery position after the seizure and wait for them to recover. They will typically have no memory of the attack and may be confused and drowsy for up to 40 minutes.

Sunburn

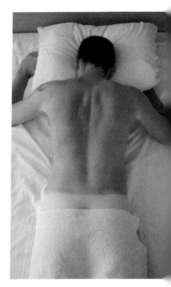

Your skin can become damaged by too much exposure to ultra violet light from the sun. Symptoms can vary in severity, depending on the length of exposure to the sun, its intensity and your skin type. Fair and freckly skinned people and red heads suffer the worst skin damage, so stay pale and mysterious!

Prevention

Common sense tips for avoiding sunburn include wearing a sunscreen with a sun protection factor of at least 15, staying out of the sun between 12 and 3 o'clock, wearing a hat and long sleeves and sitting in the shade.

Symptoms

These can include:

 Skin blisters

Swelling

Raised temperature

Redness and soreness of the skin

You may also suffer some of the symptoms associated with heatstroke (*see* below)

Treatment

Self help measures include staying out of the sun, taking a painkiller such as ibuprofen to ease inflammation, drinking lots of water and cooling the skin with a bath or shower. Applying after-sun lotion may also help. If you have severe burns or blisters you may need medical help; babies and children with skin blisters especially need urgent medical attention. Applying natural yogurt (preferably chilled in the fridge first) is a natural remedy for sunburn.

Heat Exhaustion and Heatstroke

Heat exhaustion can lead to heatstroke if left untreated. Heatstroke is a serious condition which can result in multiple organ failure and death. Both are caused by the body's thermostat overheating, causing a fall in the body's water and salt levels. Heatstroke is comparatively rare in cooler climates – apart from during heat waves, when it mainly affects older people, babies and those suffering from existing illnesses.

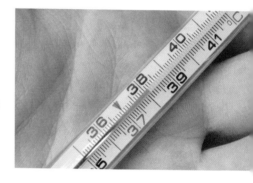

Symptoms of Heat Exhaustion

Heat exhaustion is defined as a core body temperature of between 37 and 40°C (98.6–104°F). Obviously, unless you have a thermometer to hand, you won't know this, so look out for the following symptoms:

- Skin feels hot to touch and flushed
- Profuse sweating
- Nausea/vomiting
- Fatigue
- Fainting
- Faster heart beat
- Confusion
- Producing less urine

Treatment of Heat Exhaustion

The aim of first aid treatment for heat exhaustion is to lower body temperature. The patient should recover quite quickly (within approximately 30 minutes as a rough guide), but if left untreated they may go on to develop the more serious and potentially life-threatening heatstroke (*see* below). You can help lower temperature by:

 Taking the patient to a cool place away from the sun

 Open the window or use fans or air conditioning to cool them down

 Give cool water to drink

 Sponge them down with cool water, get them to take a shower or cover them with a wet sheet

 Lay them down with their legs raised

 If possible make up a weak salt solution (approximately one teaspoon of salt to one litre of water) to speed up rehydration

 Place in recovery position and dial 999 for help if they start to deteriorate

Symptoms of Heatstroke

This is more serious and is defined as having a core body temperature of 40°C (104°F). Symptoms are similar to heat exhaustion but heatstroke patients have the following more serious symptoms too:

 Hyperventilating (rapid shallow breaths)

 Confusion

 Coordination problems

 Seizures/ fits

 Rapidly less responsive

 Loss of consciousness

Treatment

Treatment is similar to that for heat exhaustion, but you need to call for emergency medical help as soon as possible, as prompt treatment gives a much higher chance of survival. Follow the tips above for lowering body temperature and if the patient loses consciousness, check they are still breathing and that their heart is still beating. If they are not breathing then prepare to give CPR until help arrives (*see* page 226).

Overdose

Overdose can result from a deliberate or accidental overdose of drugs. The symptoms vary according to the type of drugs taken and the level of overdose:

- **Aspirin:** Overdose of aspirin can cause upper abdominal pain, nausea and vomiting, dizziness, confusion and ringing in the ears.
- **Paracetamol:** These have little noticeable effects but can cause irreversible liver damage within three days. Vomiting and nausea may develop.
- **Barbiturates and benzodiazepines:** Symptoms of overdose can include sleepiness and shallow breathing leading to unconsciousness.
- **Amphetamines (ecstasy and speed), LSD, inhaled cocaine:** Overdose signs can include sweating, hand tremor, hallucinations and hyperactive behaviour.
- **Morphine and heroin:** Symptoms of overdose can include sluggishness, mental confusion and unconsciousness.

First Aid Treatment

Try to make the patient comfortable and check vital signs. If conscious, ask what they have taken and dial 999. Search for any empty bottle, syringes etc. – the more information paramedics have the greater the chances of survival. If they are unconscious, open the airway and check breathing and give CPR if necessary (see page 226). Call 999. Do *NOT* try to make the patient vomit.

Poisoning

This happens when harmful substances or chemicals are swallowed, splashed in the eyes or on the skin, inhaled or injected (through a snake bite for instance). The body can also produce its own poisons called endotoxins or liver or kidney failure may cause poisonous substances to be produced or build up.

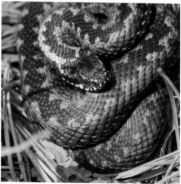

Prevention

Keep tablets and chemicals, such as bleach and dishwasher tablets, out of reach of children – particularly if you are taking children to visit relatives; older people, for example, often leave tablets out to remind them to take them.

Symptoms

These vary according to the type of poisoning but can include:

 Vomiting (sometimes containing blood)

 Unconsciousness

 Drowsiness

 Pain or burning sensation

 Drug overdose symptoms (*see* page 248)

Action and Treatment

 Call 999

 If you suspect drugs have been taken find out what they are – if they're conscious, ask them what they have taken and what quantity, or search around for chemical containers, pill packets, mushrooms and so on – and inform the emergency services

 Place them in the recovery position if they are conscious and still breathing

 Perform CPR if the casualty has stopped breathing

 Remove any clothing contaminated by chemicals

Stings and Bites

Most insect bites just cause itching and minor irritation and can be soothed by applying calamine lotion or an antihistamine cream. Bee and wasp stings whilst painful are usually not serious, unless accompanied by an anaphylactic reaction (*see* page 232). This happens to around three in 100 people – and if so you must call 999.

Symptoms

- ☑ Sharp, piercing (but short-lived) pain as the skin is pierced by the bee or wasp
- ☑ Redness
- ☑ Itching and some swelling
- ☑ Possible anaphylactic symptoms (wheezing, fast heart rate, swallowing difficulties, fainting)

Treatment

- ☑ Remove the sting as soon as possible with your fingers or tweezers, with a sideways brushing movement
- ☑ Dab with a cool clean swab
- ☑ Apply antihistamine spray to reduce inflammation
- ☑ Apply a local anaesthetic cream or spray to ease pain

Toothache

Toothache has many causes. It should never be ignored as it invariably gets worse if it isn't investigated and treated. Symptoms include:

- ☑ Pain when you chew
- ☑ Sensitivity to hot or cold food
- ☑ Bleeding around the tooth or gums
- ☑ Swelling around the tooth and/or jaw

Causes

These can include the following:

- ☑ Inflammation or infection in the middle or 'pulp' of the tooth
- ☑ Exposed tooth roots
- ☑ Dental decay
- ☑ Cracked tooth
- ☑ Sinus infection

Treatment

See a dentist, who may treat with a filling, root canal treatment or extraction. Antibiotics may be needed if an abscess has developed. Salt mouthwashes or clove oil may help. An icepack held to the face can numb the jaw and ease swelling. Simple regular painkillers such as paracetamol or ibuprofen can help.

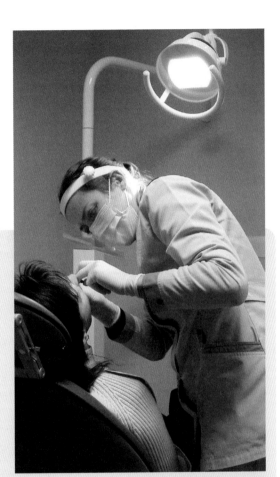

Checklist

- **Training**: Book a place on a First Aid training course.
- **Practice**: CPR techniques can be practised regularly on a dummy.
- **ABC**: Remember the ABC checklist – Airways, Breathing, Circulation.
- **Pulse**: Learn how to take a pulse.
- **Recovery position**: Memorize the recovery position.
- **Choking**: Learn how to do back blows and abdominal thrusts to clear obstructions.
- **Keep still**: Don't move someone if you suspect a spinal cord injury.
- **Adrenaline**: If you or a family member suffers severe allergies get an Epi-pen and learn how to use it.
- **Protect children**: Keep medicines and drugs out of reach of young children.

Further Reading

Banks, I., *The Man Manual: The Definitive Step-by-Step Guide to Men's Health*, J. H. Haynes & Co Ltd, 2007

Banks, I., *The Woman: A Practical Guide to Women's Health for Men*, J.H. Haynes & Co Ltd, 2004

Bean, A., *Healthy Eating for Kids*, A & C Black Publishers Ltd, 2007

Bove, Mary, N.D., *An Encyclopedia of Natural Healing for Children*, McGraw Hill/Contemporary Books, 2nd edition, 2001

Brian, K., *The Complete Guide to Female Fertility*, Piatkus, 2007

Briffa, J., *Natural Health for Kids*, Penguin, 2007

British Red Cross, *Pocket First Aid*, Dorling Kindersley, 2003

Carnegie, D., *How to Stop Worrying and Start Living*, Cedar, 1993

Courteney, H., *500 Of The Most Important Health Tips You'll Ever Need*, Cico Books, 2009

Faber, A. & Mazlish, E., *How To Talk So Kids Will Listen and Listen So Kids Will Talk*, Piccadilly Press Ltd, 2001

Harris, R. & Emberley, M., *It's Perfectly Normal: Changing Bodies, Growing Up, Sex, and Sexual Health*, Candlewick Press, 2009

Henry, J.A., *BMA New Guide to Medicine and Drugs*, Dorling Kindersley, 2007

Holford, P., *The Optimum Nutrition Bible: The Book You Have to Read If You Care About Your Health*, Piatkus, 2004

Litin, S., *Mayo Clinic Family Health Book*, HarperResource, 2003

McManners, D., *The Holistic Doctor*, Piatkus, 2004

McTaggart, L., *What Doctors Don't Tell You*, Thorsons, 2005

Siegfried, D.R., *Anatomy and Physiology for Dummies*, John Wiley & Sons, 2002

Stoppard, M., *Complete Baby and Childcare: Everything You Need to Know for the First Five Years*, Dorling Kindersley, 2008

Valman, B., *BMA When Your Child is Ill: A Home Guide for Parents*, Dorling Kindersley, 2008

Wills, J., *Feeding Kids: 120 Foolproof Family Recipes*, Headline, 2007

Websites

www.basrt.org.uk
The British Association for Sexual and Relationship Therapy (BASRT) is a specialist charity, whose members offer a range of treatments encompassing sex, psychosexual and relationship therapies.

www.bbc.co.uk/health/nutrition
The BBC's website on nutrition. Offers advice on eating a balanced diet as well as links for other informative websites and organizations.

www.bcma.co.uk
If you are interested in learning how complementary treatments can help you, or are looking for a registered practitioner, then this site is for you.

www.childrenfirst.nhs.uk
This site is by Great Ormond Street Hospital and it contains a wealth of information for children aged 4–18. It features advice, case studies and useful links.

www.eatwell.gov.uk
Offers advice on healthy diets for all stages of life. Has both a BMI calculator and a calculator that adds up how many calories an activity burns.

www.global-fitness.com/Calc.php
A calculator based on weight of a person and time spent doing an activity. Has a fairly wide variety of activities.

www.healthywomen.org.uk
Written especially for women, this site contains articles on a diverse range of issues such as the work-life balance, fertility, breastfeeding and parenting skills.

www.hhs.gov
This is the website for the US Department of Health & Human Services. If you go to the Families section you will find links to comprehensive information on how to improve the health of you and your family.

www.nhs.uk
The official site of the NHS in the UK. Helps to locate the closest GPs, hospitals, and dentists. Has health tips and a link to a page about various conditions.

www.nhsdirect.nhs.uk
Apart from listing the health line for the NHS Direct service, this website also allows you to input your symptoms to try to find a cause and information on how to proceed.

www.netfit.co.uk
An award-winning site that gives expert advice on fitness and exercise, as well and nutrition and healthy living. Offers a free motivational newsletter.

www.redcross.org.uk or **www.redcross.org**
The websites for the British and American Red Cross organization. They offer links to first aid training courses and numerous health blogs.

www.relate.org.uk
Relate offers advice, relationship counselling, sex therapy, workshops, mediation, consultations and support face-to-face, by phone and through the website.

www.sja.org.uk
The official site for St John Ambulance. Offers links to first aid training courses. Also gives advice on first aid in different situations.

www.supernanny.co.uk
Compiled by experts, this super site contains loads of practical tips and advice on how to be a better parent. Includes downloadable reward charts, forums and more.

www.webmd.com
This site offers advice on various aspects of health, from healthy living and eating to different drugs. It also allows a person to self-diagnose based on symptoms – in order to be discussed with a physician, not as final diagnoses.

Index